SAY WHY TO DRUGS

Everything You Need to Know About the
Drugs We Take and Why We Get High

Dr Suzi Gage

HODDER &
STOUGHTON

First published in Great Britain in 2020 by Hodder & Stoughton
An Hachette UK company

1

A CIP catalogue record for this title is available from the British Library

Hardback ISBN 9781473686229
Trade Paperback ISBN 9781473686236
eBook ISBN 9781473686250

Typeset in Adobe Caslon by
Palimpsest Book Production Ltd, Falkirk, Stirlingshire

Printed and bound in Great Britain by
Clays Ltd, Elcograf S.p.A.

Hodder & Stoughton policy is to use papers that are natural, renewable
and recyclable products and made from wood grown in sustainable forests.
The logging and manufacturing processes are expected to conform
to the environmental regulations of the country of origin.

Hodder & Stoughton Ltd
Carmelite House
50 Victoria Embankment
London EC4Y 0DZ

www.hodder.co.uk

For L

Contents

Foreword

You are not entitled to your opinion.
You are entitled to your informed opinion.
No one is entitled to be ignorant.
HARLAN ELLISON

The internet has given us access to so much information and provided us with the ability to have an opinion on such a wide variety of subjects . . . but we seem to focus heavily on the latter and not so much on the former.

Drugs are one such topic. People love to have an opinion, but the waters are so muddied with fearmongering and bias that it is hard to figure out how to inform that opinion reliably. It is for this reason that I am so overwhelmingly proud for even the small part I have played in helping *Say Why to Drugs* to exist.

Way back in 2015, it was the internet that made me aware of Dr Suzi Gage and led to her becoming a guest on my *Distraction Pieces Podcast*. In that very first recorded conversation, the seeds were watered for the idea of a podcast that provided an unbiased, fact-based education on the taboo subject of drugs. Not getting mixed up in the opinion and often emotion-led argument of 'right or wrong / good or evil', but simply focusing on facts and studies.

I had just begun working on the idea of using the reach of my podcast to expand and build a network of podcasts, giving a platform to people I felt were more than deserving of one. As you can imagine, I was keen for one of the first additions to the network to be the realisation of Suzi's podcast ideas.

At this stage, I was already starting to worry that, as podcasts were growing, the quote that opened this foreword was getting more and more ignored. So many opinions, so few informed ones. Thus, having suggested the name *Say Why to Drugs* to Suzi, I was even more motivated to do anything I could to help bring a researched, informed and rational podcast on a much-mythologised subject to the ever-growing podcast world.

When Suzi was ready to launch, she decided it would work best, format wise, if she had a guest on each episode to discuss it all with her. What better way to confirm or dispel a myth than for it to be presented by someone who believes it and addressed by someone who has studied it? I was lucky enough to be asked to be that said guest.

As the episodes went on, Suzi decided that I was a good fit to have a regular position as the guest for a few reasons. The clearest reason was that, in my youth, I had tried a fair number of the drugs in question and was happy to discuss openly my experiences. I feel it also helped that, through nothing but personal choice, I now do not take any drugs apart from the occasional drop of alcohol – and I truly mean occasional, as I tend to drink only eight or nine times a year.

This was all well and good and to be involved felt great . . . but it was the reaction when it launched that was truly overwhelming.

Listenership exceeded all expectation and feedback was coming in from parents and teachers who wished that they had had such a resource when they were in their younger, experimental years. Young and old, those who had used drugs and those that had not, the podcast seemed to reach so many people. People who needed to hear it.

And now it's a book!

A real-life actual book that you are reading.

I truly believe that what Suzi has created here will live on as an essential tool in the 'war on ignorance'; the natural successor and antidote to start repairing the damage done by the 'war on drugs'.

Scroobius Pip
July 2019

Introduction

Have you ever taken drugs?

Every time I ask this question as part of a talk or lecture, a few people put their hands up. And sometimes, when these talks are at events like *Skeptics in the Pub*, I then mischievously point out that the pint of beer in front of them contains a psychoactive substance. Almost all of us have at least tried a psychoactive substance, from our cuppa in the morning, to a teenage coughing fit after a cigarette behind the bike sheds, or a vodka-filled alcopop, even if we decide not to try them again, or have never tried anything 'illicit'.

If you have tried drugs (and I have, I'm sipping a coffee as I write this), you are not alone. Humans have been enjoying the effects of psychoactive substances for thousands of years. If chewing a particular leaf might improve your concentration, speed or accuracy, you might be more likely to catch and therefore eat meat that day – it's clear why that would have been advantageous.

Psychoactive drugs have also been used in ritualistic settings for centuries – shamans imbibing psychedelic substances to allow them to communicate with gods or spirits. Tobacco and cannabis were both initially used in ritualistic settings. Psychedelic drugs such as ayahuasca still are in some Amazonian communities.

The UK's drug of choice, alcohol, has probably been around since the Stone Age. Some historians believe that alcohol was a food staple before bread, as it contained plenty of carbo-hydrates. In all likelihood, it was considerably weaker than the beers we're used to today – evidence suggests that even children drank it.

What about more recently? Fast forward to the turn of the last century, when machine rolling of cigarettes meant they could be mass-produced, and we see a new way to consume tobacco. In the UK and USA, the inclusion of cigarettes in soldiers' ration packs during the First and Second World Wars really cemented their place as a drug of choice in the countries. And even though cigarettes have fallen out of favour more recently, as evidence of how much of a health risk they are has weakened their appeal, the World Health Organisation estimate that as of 2018 there are still 1.1 billion smokers worldwide, with 6.1 million of them in the UK.

Even more Brits drink alcohol – around 58 per cent of UK adults (those over sixteen) drank alcohol in the previous week, according to the Office for National Statistics. And the history of alcohol as the UK's drug of choice is long and rich.

As would be expected, illicit drugs are not as widely used. According to the European Monitoring Centre for Drugs and Drug Addiction (EMCDDA) 2019 report, just under 10 per cent of UK adults (which they define as those aged between sixteen and fifty-nine) have used an illicit substance in the past year. Cannabis is the most commonly used; the same report found that 12.3 per cent of sixteen- to thirty-four-year-olds in the UK reported using cannabis in the past year. Other drugs are even less common – cocaine use was reported by roughly 5 per cent of those surveyed, and MDMA by 3 per cent.

Drug-use patterns are surprisingly inconsistent across the world. In East Asia, amphetamines are the illicit drug of choice. Alcohol is less popular than in the West, in part due to genetic differences that result in a reduction in ability to metabolise alcohol in a significant proportion of the population, leaving some people with unpleasant flushing and nausea symptoms if they drink even a small amount.

In Germany, like the UK, cannabis is the most commonly used illicit drug. The next most common are amphetamines, although these are being used by less than 2 per cent of the population. In some countries, particular drug-use patterns occur because drugs are trafficked through them. For example, there's a distinct increase in opioid use in countries that lie between Afghanistan, where the poppies are grown, and western Europe and the USA, where opiates can be sold for big money. In Russia, one route used to traffic heroin to Europe, HIV cases have shot up in recent years, with around half of new cases linked to injecting drug use.

But although the drug of choice may be different, there doesn't seem to be any culture where drug use in some form or another hasn't been documented or observed. There seems to be something about humans that makes us want to alter our perception in some way. Is drug use innate? I am not sure, but anthropologist Donald E. Brown certainly believes it's important – he listed 'mood- or consciousness-altering techniques or substances' as a 'human universal', something found in all societies and cultures, ranking psychoactive substance use alongside music, language and play.

Drugs have inspired works of art throughout history, from novels and plays to paintings and movies. The evocative *Gin Lane* by William Hogarth, depicting perhaps a scaremongering vision of gin-addled London in the mid-1700s, might even be considered the first public health advert, as it was created to support a proposed Gin Act that was an attempt to curb drinking in the city, and contrasted with its sister piece, the far more wholesomely portrayed *Beer Street*.

Legality may also have an influence on the prevalence of drug use, but not necessarily in the way you might suspect. In Portugal, for example, where drug use was decriminalised in 2001, prevalence of illicit drug use is much lower than most of the rest of

Europe. The EMCDDA report puts cannabis use among young people in the last year at around 5 per cent, with cocaine, MDMA and amphetamines all being used by less than 1 per cent of the population.

I will use the terms 'psychoactive substances' and 'drugs' throughout this book, but these can be quite difficult terms to define. Drugs can mean medication we are prescribed by our doctors or substances we take for recreation, and the two aren't necessarily mutually exclusive. Ketamine, opiates, even cannabis all have medical uses, and trials investigating therapeutic properties of MDMA and psilocybin, the active compound in magic mushrooms, are ongoing.

The UK government introduced the 'psychoactive substances bill' in 2016 and defined the term as something that 'by stimulating or depressing the person's nervous system . . . affects the person's mental functioning or emotional state'.

Think about the way a glass of wine can make you feel relaxed, and two or three can affect your ability to think clearly. (This definition isn't that brilliant, though – chocolate or sweets, maybe even sex, could legitimately be defined by the description above.) Some psychoactive substances, like alcohol and tobacco, are legal, while others are not, although that wasn't always the case. Cannabis and opium, for example, have a complicated history in terms of their legality and corresponding social acceptability.

Taking any psychoactive substance is not without risk. Most, if not all, of the substances we take to alter our brain do so in a way that makes them potentially psychologically or physically addictive. Whether addiction in and of itself is harmful is a topic we'll get on to, but there are other risks, too. Most psychoactive substances also impact on the body – stimulants increase heart rate and blood pressure, which can put a strain on the heart and circulatory system, while depressants can slow things down (like breathing) and potentially lead to loss of consciousness, or worse.

Tolerance can also build up, meaning more of the drug needs to be consumed to get the same effect. And longer-term risks to health are possible as well. We all know the greatly increased risk of lung cancer and other diseases that cigarette use causes. But maybe other drugs are having other, albeit less extreme, effects. Does MDMA use really lead to depression? Can too much cannabis cause schizophrenia? These are much harder questions to answer, so the information that reaches the mainstream media about these questions is much more difficult to follow.

I have been fascinated by the science around the use of recreational drugs since I was an undergraduate psychology student at UCL way back in the early 2000s. But I have a particular interest in the link between drug use and mental health. I did my PhD in Bristol, looking at the links between cannabis and cigarette use, and later depressive symptoms or psychotic-like experiences, by studying a group of UK-based teenagers called Children of the 90s, who have had data collected on them since before they were born.

I'm a psychologist (although a researcher rather than a clinical psychologist) and an epidemiologist – I now work at the University of Liverpool, where I teach medical students and do my own research. But I'm not a medical doctor. As such, when I present evidence, I'm talking about research evidence, often at a population level. This book aims to provide information about recreational drugs, based on scientific evidence. It's not a political book – it is not an argument for or against legalisation or regulation of substances. It's trying to be as dispassionate as possible and sticking only to what we've uncovered through scientific research.

This means there will be times when I'll tell you that we don't know the answer – I hope that is OK. But one thing I will do my utmost to avoid is the addition of any hyperbole, any spin, or any judgment. However, I can't promise that I won't sneak in any stealth statistics lessons. And here's the first, about how it's so difficult to do research looking at drugs.

When we do population science, epidemiology* as it's known, we often want to find out whether a particular behaviour or environmental exposure increases or decreases the risk of some negative (or positive) outcome. The best way to do this would be to conduct what's called a randomised controlled trial. Say you're interested in finding out whether taking vitamin supplements is associated with the risk of getting a cold. You'd take a large group of individuals (and I mean large, we're talking hundreds or, ideally, thousands here), and randomly assign half to receive the vitamin, and half to receive a placebo sugar pill.

In order to minimise bias, you wouldn't tell the individual in question whether they were getting vitamin or placebo, and the experimenter wouldn't know until after the data had been collected either. The people enrolled in the study would be followed up for an appropriate length of time, and the number of people getting colds in each group would be calculated and statistically tested to work out the likelihood that any differences seen could have occurred by chance.

You see the problem here when we're talking about substance use. Despite my best attempts at persuading university ethics committees,† they're not really keen on us recruiting a bunch of teenagers and randomly asking one group to smoke, one to drink alcohol, and another to start using cannabis, even if we could persuade them to stick to only one substance throughout the trial, which given teenagers' proclivity for risk-taking behaviour, being led by their peers, and experimentation, is unlikely.

Because we can't do an experiment, we are left to observe what people choose to do. And the people who choose to use cannabis

---

* Epidemiology comes from the same root as epidemic (rather than epidermis – I have had people ask me a number of times if I do work investigating the skin).

† I am, of course, joking – this would be a horrendous unethical and impractical experiment to run.

(as an example) are likely to be different from people who choose not to in loads of other ways – they might also be more likely to drink alcohol or smoke cigarettes, there might be differences in their childhood experiences that led some of them to experiment with cannabis, or in their peer groups (if your friends are all using it, you might be more likely to try it, simply because you have access to it). We try to take these differences into account using statistical techniques, but this relies on two factors: knowing what all the differences are, and being able to measure them accurately.

Because of these limitations, it's very difficult to be sure that an association means one thing causes the other. If we see depression at higher levels in people who drink alcohol than those who don't, does that mean that alcohol increases the risk of depression, or that having depression leads to people being more likely to start drinking, or to drink more heavily? A third option is that some other factor (struggling at work maybe, or going through a divorce) might increase both the risk of depression and the likelihood to drink.

As the cliché goes, correlation does not equal causation . . . except when it does, of course, but that's not every time. So how do we work out which scenario is correct? Throughout this book I'll try and pull out useful ways of interpreting studies you might see reported in the newspaper, and I will consider what makes certain study designs better or worse in terms of providing good evidence.

Given that drug use might be a 'human universal' – it's been seen throughout history, and most of us have at the very least dabbled, or know someone who has – it is worrying how much misinformation there is about how drugs affect the brain and body, and the potential risks of using them. And for a small but important minority, the risks of taking drugs can be severe. Do we know who is at risk? Are there ways of predicting it, and preventing it?

This is a book that you can sit and read from cover to cover, but equally if there are particular substances you're interested in, it's also fine to dip into any chapter, and flick back and forth through the book. To help with that, I've also added a glossary at the end of the book, so I won't define terms every time they crop up.

For each substance in the book, we'll cover the short-term intoxication effects and potential long-term risks from regular use of the substance, we'll tackle the myths and misconceptions that exist around them, and whether they have any medical uses, as well as covering all sorts of interesting findings, history and cutting-edge research that is currently going on. Where I've interviewed individuals about their drug use, some names have been changed.

You have probably heard a number of the categories that recreational drugs fall into. Stimulants, depressants, hallucinogens, uppers, downers . . . all sorts of terms get bandied about, but what do they mean? What's the difference between a stimulant and a hallucinogen? Throughout the book, I will also be interspersing mini-chapters that give the low-down on what these terms mean, which drugs fall into which categories, and the key characteristics that those substances have.

In this book there won't be any judgment, there won't be any hyperbole, there will be (a few) stats. Are you ready? Let's go.

CHAPTER 1

Alcohol

What is it? Fermented from fruit or grains, alcohol (ethanol) can be found as beer, wine or spirits.

Type of drug: A depressant, but can seem to have stimulant effects at low doses.

Popularity: Globally extremely popular, legal in most countries, although some religions do not permit alcohol consumption.

How consumed: Drunk (which is also how you'll end up).

Timescale: Peak intoxication 45–90 mins after consumption.

Some effects: Sociability, lowering of inhibitions, loss of motor control, impaired judgment.

WHEN WE TALK about alcohol as a recreational drug, we really mean ethanol, a particular type of alcohol that is produced when sugar is fermented by yeast. Alcoholic drinks are usually made from fermented fruits or grains, and broadly fall into three categories: beers, wines, and spirits. Alcoholic drinks have a long history of use across the globe, from Stone Age beer jugs to

Ancient Egyptian brewing and Babylonian wine deities, and they are very much ingrained in many cultures worldwide. Ale was extremely popular in the Middle Ages in the UK, though it was much weaker, and consumed daily in large quantities, potentially by all ages.

While underage drinking is discouraged these days, alcohol is still very much part of British culture. Office of National Statistics figures from 2017 found that only 16 per cent of white adults in Great Britain reported being teetotal, although the figure was around 50 per cent for other ethnicities. But while alcohol remains the drug of choice in the UK and in much of Judaeo–Christian culture, there's some suggestion that this is changing.

Certainly in the UK, and indeed in many Western cultures around the globe, there is one group of people in whom drinking rates are going down. And it's not necessarily the group you'd expect. In fact, it's young people, defined as those aged twenty-five or younger in most places. For this group, national statistics suggest that the number of drinking occasions in a given month is lower than it's ever been, and there is a larger proportion of teetotallers in this group than at any time since data began being collected.

At present, it's not really clear why we're seeing this drop in alcohol use in young people. Perhaps this group spend their time differently than the same age-group did in the 1990s or 2000s – preferring to socialise online, at home, or maybe even worried that drunken photos will be uploaded online before you can say 'Instagram'. Perhaps public-health messages about the harms of drinking are hitting home. Maybe young people are rebelling against the heavy drinking of their parents' generation.

In all probability it's unlikely that any one factor will be solely responsible. It may even be a statistical anomaly – what goes up must come down, and alcohol use in young adults was at its highest around the year 2000, so perhaps this fall is to be expected in the ebb and flow of population health behaviours. It's hard to say. And just because young people are drinking less regularly, doesn't mean they aren't still partaking in dangerous drinking patterns.

When young people are drinking, they are still reporting binge drinking – drinking to the point of illness, well above recommended levels. In fact, the 2017 ONS report mentioned above found that while young people aged sixteen to twenty-four years old were less likely to drink than any other age group in Great Britain, they also found that when they did drink, they were drinking more on a given day than any other age group. But what does alcohol do to us when we drink it?

What are the short-term effects?

Many people reading this are probably familiar with the symptoms of alcohol intoxication. I know I am. Alcohol takes between ten minutes to an hour to get into the bloodstream, and its effects vary depending on the dose. It might take forty-five to ninety minutes to feel the peak effect of a drink once it has been consumed. After an average drink, you might feel more sociable and warm – the feeling described as 'tipsy'. At this level of alcohol consumption your heart rate has increased, and your blood vessels have dilated. Your inhibitions might be slightly lowered, too, and you might feel relaxed.

As you drink more alcohol, the effects get more pronounced. You can start to feel lightheaded, and you might struggle with fine motor tasks (ever tried threading a needle while drunk? Or trying to unlock your front door?). As well as these physical effects, your judgment and decision making can become impaired. This is why drinking in moderation can be so difficult – it's easy when sober to decide that one or two drinks is all you're going to have that evening, but once you've had those drinks – even just one or two – you might feel less concerned with your plans for the next morning, and more keen to carry on the night.

If you do continue drinking beyond this point, things can get worse. You might experience memory blackouts, you could end up nauseous and vomiting, your motor control will get worse, potentially leading to stumbles and falls, and this, combined with impaired judgment, can lead to serious accidents.

There's some evidence that alcohol intoxication might increase aggression, but at the moment it's pretty weak. What might explain the fights that seem to occur more often among intoxicated people could be an increase in misinterpreting ambiguous emotional faces. If you see a person with a neutral expression when you're sober, you probably think nothing of it, but while drunk, you might misinterpret that lack of a smile as aggression. And if that person is drunk too, that misinterpretation could escalate. Or maybe it's due to a lowering of barriers that keep us conforming to social niceties and expectations.

Intoxication is also associated with increased risk of sexually transmitted diseases and unplanned pregnancies – when we're drunk, we are more likely to partake in risky behaviours, and this can include unprotected sex, as well as fights.

Within the brain, alcohol affects almost every neurotransmitter that we have. These are the chemicals that transmit signals between our brain cells. Different neurotransmitters are associated with different pathways or networks in the brain, so manipulating particular ones will lead to particular effects – on bodily functions, ability to think, motor skills, even emotion or mood. Alcohol is often referred to as a global or 'dirty' drug, and it's this effect on so many different neurotransmitters that can make it appear like a stimulant or a depressant depending on the dose and time after drinking.

For some people, the consumption of alcohol, even at low levels, can be really unpleasant. And this is down to genetics. Small caveat: it's very rare that one particular genetic variant or gene is responsible for a big change in behaviour (called a pheno-type in this field of research), but this is one of those unusual examples.* In populations of European descent,† a broad defini-tion of which includes most people native to Europe and North America, this atypical version of the gene is extremely rare. However, in people with East Asian heritage, it's much more common, with estimates that around one-third to one-half of these populations have at least one copy of the atypical gene, or even two – one inherited from each parent.

So what does this gene do, and why is it a problem to have an atypical version? The gene codes for an enzyme called aldehyde dehydrogenase. This enzyme is the second step of alcohol break-down from ethanol into acetic acid, which the body can excrete. In the first step, alcohol gets broken down by another enzyme (alcohol dehydrogenase) into acetaldehyde. Acetaldehyde is not very nice, it's pretty toxic, and it's one of the chemicals that has been blamed for the nausea we can feel when really drunk or hung over.

For people with the atypical gene, and the faulty enzyme, their bodies break down alcohol into acetaldehyde, but then the faulty aldehyde dehydrogenase enzyme can't break this down any further, so unpleasant levels of it build up in the body. The upshot of this is that the individual feels sick, sweaty, headachy, and their face will flush red. As such, many people with one or two of these atypical variants will avoid alcohol altogether – which is one of the reasons that problematic alcohol use, and alcohol-related cancers are rarer in East Asian populations than in European populations.

---

* As a rule of thumb, if you see a headline saying 'gene for x discovered', it's almost always not the case.

† The genetics of race is extremely complicated and contentious, so here I'm talking in broad strokes about population averages – there's actually not very good evidence for meaningful systematic genetic differences between races.

Some people describe the experience of drinking with an atypical aldehyde dehydrogenase gene as like 'an instant hangover'. But what actually is a hangover? In very simple terms, it's the awful feeling we can experience the morning (or day . . . or entire week – not that I'm speaking from experience, you understand) after a heavy night of drinking alcohol. This can include being unable to move more than a few feet from the loo in case you're sick; a pounding headache that's sensitive to noise, light and even smell; aching joints, and for some people a feeling of anxiety or sadness.

Yet despite this being something that many of us will have experienced, there's surprisingly little research into why we get hangovers, and whether there's anything we can do to minimise the symptoms.

Recently, work was published that somewhat disproved the old maxim 'Beer before wine, feel fine. Wine before beer, feel queer.' In a sample of ninety individuals, hangover severity was not affected by the order in which different alcoholic drinks were presented. There is, however, some evidence that the type of drink consumed could impact on a hangover. Alcohol that is darker in colour tends to contain more compounds called congeners, and there's some evidence from the 1970s that suggested that congener-heavy alcohol, like brandy or red wine, led to more risk of hangover than clear spirits like gin or vodka.

This area of research was recently updated, and researchers found that while individuals reported feeling worse after consuming bourbon (compared to vodka), when they were tested on a number of metrics including sleep, memory and reaction times, there was no difference between the groups. There are a number of research groups who have recently started looking in more depth into the hangover and its effect on us.

One is led by Dr Sally Adams at the University of Bath. She and her team recently published a paper that systematically reviewed all the research published to date that investigated the impact of a hangover on cognition. They found nineteen research papers that had investigated this question, and concluded that the evidence to date suggests we're likely to be impaired in our ability to perform tasks that require sustained attention not only while we're drunk, but the next day as well. They also found evidence that a hangover might impact on our ability to drive – so even after we'd pass a breathalyser test, we might want to think twice before getting behind the wheel if we're feeling wretched.

What are the longer-term effects?

Long-term alcohol use is known to increase the risk of liver problems. Heavy drinking, even in the short term, can lead to a build-up of fat in the liver, which is a reversible warning sign of alcohol-related liver disease. If the liver isn't given a break from alcohol to recover, more serious disease can set in, with symptoms often not being seen until the liver is substantially damaged.

There is a large body of evidence causally linking alcohol to seven types of cancer, including breast cancer, liver cancer, mouth cancer and bowel cancer. The charity Cancer Research UK have stated that alcohol is responsible for approximately 4 per cent of UK cancer diagnoses. As an example, people who drink one typical alcoholic drink a day have an estimated 20-per-cent increased risk of mouth cancer compared to those who don't drink at all. Which sounds like a massive increase, but mouth cancer is fairly rare – around five in 1,000 non-drinkers will develop mouth cancer at some point in their life, and a 20-per-cent increased risk roughly equates to one more diagnosis of cancer per 1,000 individuals.

Heavier drinking increases your risk more – if everyone drank at least 44 units a week (about four and a half bottles of wine), that would result in eleven extra cases of mouth cancer per 1,000 individuals, on top of the baseline five. This illustrates the difference between what's called a 'relative risk' and an 'absolute risk'.

Describing something as a 'twenty-per-cent increased risk' is a relative risk – and these are often the figures the media will report as they sound really dramatic. But if you as an individual want to make an informed choice about whether to do something or not, the absolute risk is far more informative. Relative risks can look massive, but if the underlying risk is extremely low then increasing it by 20 per cent, even 50 per cent, will still result in a low, albeit ever-so-slightly higher risk.

Alcohol can be dependence forming – about 9 per cent of men and 4 per cent of women in the UK show symptoms of alcohol dependence. However, the term 'alcoholic' to describe people with alcohol dependence is falling out of favour among many researchers, clinicians and policy makers. While some in the past have said that defining alcohol problems as the disease 'alcoholism' can shift stigma away from an individual, others fear that such labels are equally stigmatising, implying 'rock bottom' and a lifelong diagnosis.

As well as this, the term might create an 'othering' of problematic alcohol use, giving some people something like a get-out clause – 'Oh well, my drinking isn't as bad at *that*, I'm not an alcoholic so I don't need to do anything about my drinking.' Problematic alcohol use exists on a spectrum, and people can improve their relationship with alcohol even if they haven't yet reached a severe problem.

All this isn't to say that the term is not useful to an individual – I have met a number of people who self-identify as an 'alcoholic', and some told me that it helps them in terms of maintaining their abstinence from alcohol and avoiding relapse. However, they also said that self-identifying as an alcoholic is worlds away from being labelled an alcoholic by other people, or society. As with other addictions (and this is explored in more detail in the Addiction chapter), stigma is high towards people with alcohol-use disorder, which can impact their recovery, their ability to find employment, and all sorts of aspects of their lives.

Alcohol tolerance builds up over time, meaning a person needs to consume more alcohol to get the same effect, and it can be a struggle to cut down even when a person has health problems. There are also physical withdrawal symptoms when trying to quit alcohol, and these can include seizures and can potentially be extremely dangerous. Also, as alcohol tolerance will reduce if a person abstains, overdosing on alcohol during relapse is easily done and can have severe, even fatal, consequences.

Long-term alcohol use can impact negatively on an individual's mental health. It has been linked to increased risk of depression and anxiety, to memory impairment, and to increased levels of stress. Although, as with other substances, understanding the links with mental health is more challenging than for physical health. And yet, many people will use alcohol as a method of managing their anxiety. In particular, social anxiety – I'm sure lots of us have done this.

Imagine you have to go to a party, perhaps organised by a friend of a friend. You're not going to know anyone there, you're not going to like the music, and you'd really rather not go. In this circumstance, many people would use alcohol to make the party more bearable. For those with more severe anxiety, perhaps untreated, alcohol can seem like an easy and socially acceptable method for self-medication. It's even marketed as such – 'keep calm and drink prosecco', 'mummy needs her gin' – and this appears particularly to be the case where women are concerned. But using alcohol in this way, sometimes referred to as 'drinking to cope', is likely to be maladaptive.

As I mentioned earlier, alcohol use is associated with an increased risk of depression and anxiety. So while in the short-term a drink or two might help with your current situation, in the long run it might be making things worse. Set and setting are important here. Alcohol intoxication will be affected by where you are, and your state of mind. If you are unhappy or anxious and you start drinking, you might initially feel better, but this could easily end up with you feeling awful and crying in the toilets (I speak from painful experience here).

Can alcohol be good for you?

You've probably at some point seen headlines saying a glass of red wine is good for you. Sadly, the evidence doesn't really back this up. There have been a few studies of a chemical called resveratrol, which is found in red grape skins (and therefore in red wine). In animal studies and cell-culture studies, this chemical has been linked to benefits for diabetes, neurodegenerative diseases and even cancer. However, scaling this up to humans has been challenging, because the quantity of resveratrol you'd have to consume is enormous, and consuming that dose, even in trials of extracted resveratrol, has been very difficult.

This doesn't mean that resveratrol doesn't have any beneficial effects, but at the moment we simply don't have enough evidence. And, of course, resveratrol isn't the only chemical in red wine, and we know that alcohol causes seven types of cancer. So to say that red wine might be beneficial for cancer is just plain wrong.

More controversial are the findings that suggest a beneficial effect of drinking a small amount of alcohol, compared to none, in particular around risk for heart disease or stroke. There is some disagreement in academic circles around this so-called 'J'-shaped curve. Looking at these graphs, it seems to indicate that not drinking any alcohol at all is more dangerous than drinking a small amount. But plenty of academics are sceptical about this.

As we've already discussed, not drinking any alcohol at all is surprisingly rare. And the people who choose not to drink anything are different from the people who drink a small amount. I know that when I'm unwell, I'm less keen to drink alcohol, so it's plausible that if I had a long-term illness, I might stop drinking altogether. People might also be advised, if their health is poor, to stop drinking by their doctor.

Another group of people who don't drink at all are those managing alcohol dependence. Some people choose not to drink alcohol for religious reasons. And there are loads of other people who don't drink – who come from all walks of life. Not everyone who doesn't drink is likely to have poor health, but if enough do, that is likely to skew any findings.

It's not surprising that people who drink a lot of alcohol have an increased risk of health problems of all kinds. So what about these people who drink a small amount and seem to be the most healthy? Well, perhaps they're just the healthiest group to begin with. Maybe they do the most exercise, are the most well off, or eat the most healthily.

These sound like generalisations, and they absolutely are. There will be people who fit all those descriptions who don't drink anything, and people who have long-term illnesses who drink a small amount of alcohol. But when we do observational studies we look 'at the population level', so it's about the majority.

This is again a problem with using observational cohort studies – people who don't drink at all are 'on the whole' different from people who drink a small amount, and accounting for these differences is difficult. It's also why we get anomalies like the 80-year-old-granny-who-smokes-like-a-chimney that everyone seems to know. We're always talking about differences in risk at the level of a whole population, rather than for an individual.

But there is one way in which alcohol is extremely beneficial for health, and in fact you've probably encountered it every time you've been to a hospital. Not to drink, though – alcohol hand sanitiser is extremely effective at reducing the spread of bacteria and germs.

And we drink it.

For fun.

More curiously, alcohol does seem to have some other unusual effects that could potentially be seen as being good for us. Some of my former colleagues at the University of Bristol have found some really interesting results, when they brought people into the lab and asked them to consume alcohol. After doing this, they got the intoxicated people to rate the attractiveness of faces of the same gender, the opposite gender, and some images of landscapes. As might be expected, the so-called 'beer goggles' effect was found – intoxicated individuals rated all stimuli as more attractive than people who'd been given a placebo non-alcoholic drink did.

However, when the same researchers followed up their findings in a naturalistic environment (they took their stimuli and a breathalyser into a local pub), they weren't able to replicate these findings. Does that mean the beer goggles effect is a myth? Maybe, although the levels of alcohol in the pub setting were on the lower end of intoxicated, and the effect has previously been found to increase with dose.

But still, this says something interesting about how we conduct experiments on alcohol. Often these are done in a lab in a university department. A participant coming in and being given alcohol, then asked to rate a load of faces might be primed to 'please' the experimenter – however hard we try and avoid this through clever or thoughtful study designs. And these kinds of designs are not really representative of how we drink in the real world. Drinking is often (though not always) a social occasion, and rarely something we do sitting on our own in a university building.

Which is not to say that there isn't value in conducting lab studies. And some universities have novel ways to get around this problem. At the University of Liverpool, where I work, researchers have built a bespoke 'bar lab' in the psychology department. It's an amazing space, decked out to look like a bar or a pub, but with the ability to control the surrounding environment to increase consistency, something that it's much harder to do when you take a study out into the real world!

More recently, the group in Bristol have continued their research into alcohol and attractiveness and found something really surprising. They brought people into the lab and gave them varying quantities of alcohol. But rather than asking them to rate the attractiveness of other people, they took their photograph before and after alcohol. They then showed these pairs of photos to other people, and found that how intoxicated an individual is will impact on how attractive other people find them.

A small amount of alcohol (roughly equivalent to one glass of wine) was associated with the highest ratings of attractiveness. Any more alcohol than this and the effect went away, but I find this finding completely fascinating. There's a lot of research from evolutionary psychology that has indicated that skin tone impacts on rates of attractiveness. Perhaps the mild flush in a person's cheeks after alcohol can lead to this subtle effect. Perhaps a person is more relaxed (or maybe less inhibited is a more accurate way of phrasing this) after a small amount of alcohol and so is more at ease in front of the camera.

It's impossible to say from these findings, but it might be another part of the puzzle that explains why increased levels of risky sexual behaviour are seen after alcohol intoxication. The heady mix of lower inhibitions, potentially finding others more attractive, and looking more attractive yourself could be quite the cocktail of risk behaviours!

What don't we know?

There's still a surprisingly large list of things we know little about regarding our drug of choice. For example, we know that alcohol is a teratogen – that is, it can cause damage to a developing foetus – but how the risk of consuming a very small amount of alcohol during pregnancy is less clear. At the moment the guidelines in the UK recommend avoiding alcohol if trying to conceive, and during pregnancy. And we know that regular drinking while pregnant can lead to foetal alcohol syndrome, and that there is more of a spectrum of foetal alcohol effects than previously thought, meaning even a moderate amount of alcohol could impact on the foetus. A recent systematic review concluded that even though evidence was sparse, there were some studies that found an association with preterm delivery and smaller babies even at very low levels of alcohol consumption during pregnancy. These outcomes are themselves risk factors for other negative outcomes in childhood, suggesting that any alcohol during pregnancy should be avoided wherever possible. Of course, if a woman has gone out drinking and then finds out she is pregnant, it is not true that there will have been damage caused to the child. And it is important that women and healthcare professionals are able to have honest, judgment-free conversations to ensure adequate support to make the rest of her pregnancy alcohol free, rather than a woman feeling stressed and guilty when she finds out she is pregnant and potentially not wanting to speak to her healthcare provider about this. That said, the sparse evidence we have to date suggests the precautionary principle endorsed by the UK guidelines at present is sensible advice, for women who are planning a pregnancy, and for those who are already pregnant.

CHAPTER 2

Amphetamine

What is it? Synthesised powder or pill.
Type of drug: Stimulant.
Popularity: Southeast Asia and Australasia in particular.
How consumed: Swallowed, snorted, smoked or injected.
Timescale: Varies with consumption method – 4 to 8 hours.
Some effects: Increased confidence, alertness, heart rate,
  blood pressure, body temperature.

WHETHER YOU'VE SEEN *Breaking Bad*, or you've read about speed freaks in Beat poetry from the 1950s, amphetamine has a rich cultural history. And the substance also has a long medical history. Amphetamine was first synthesised in the late 1800s, but it wasn't patented or investigated as a medication until the 1930s. It was synthesised as an attempt to improve on a substance called ephedrine, which was used at the time as a treatment for asthma.

Ephedrine had a number of side-effects, including trouble

sleeping, anxiety, hallucinations, even risk of stroke or heart attack. It was also prone to abuse. Amphetamine was chemically similar to ephedrine, and the hope was that it would not have these side-effects. While amphetamine wasn't a brilliant treatment for asthma, inhalers containing it were marketed as Benzedrine, both for asthma and as a nasal decongestant. Even now, ephedrine and pseudoephedrine remain in some over-the-counter nasal decongestant sprays.

Amphetamine's stimulant properties were also noticed during research on the compound, and during the Second World War amphetamine pills were used by British and American troops, while German and Japanese forces were taking the chemically similar analogue methamphetamine. Amphetamine as a medication to treat depression fell somewhat out of favour when other, less dependence-forming medications were developed, but it is still prescribed to this day, now as a treatment for attention deficit hyperactivity disorder (ADHD – the medication branded as Adderall contains d-amphetamine and a small amount of levoamphetamine).

Amphetamine has been popular as a diet pill, as a means to stay awake or alert, and as a study aid (while we might think of the use of chemical cognitive enhancers as something modern, the first media reports of students (mis)using amphetamine to help them study came way back in 1937, the same year it was first marketed).

Amphetamine is particularly popular in Asia, Australasia, and North America, and overall it has historically been the second most widely used illicit drug worldwide, after cannabis. I say historically, as the World Drug Report from the UN Office on Drugs and Crime, published in 2018, found that opioid use is now equal to amphetamine use worldwide, with an estimated 34 million individuals using either substance at least once in 2016.

What is it?

The term 'amphetamine' is often used as a catch-all for substances including amphetamine sulphate and methamphetamine. These are chemically very similar, although methamphetamine absorbs more easily into fats – a quality known as lipophilia.

Amphetamine sulphate is a stimulant – it's sometimes known as speed or whiz,* but you might also have heard of the brand names Benzadrine or Adderall. It can be a white/off white or pinkish crystal powder, it can be in pill form, or it is sometimes found as a putty-like substance. It can also be found in a freebase form (similar to the differences between cocaine and crack cocaine), which is an oily liquid.

Methamphetamine is chemically similar to amphetamine, but is more potent, and can cross the blood-brain barrier more quickly. Methamphetamine is often called meth, crystal meth, or ice. Meth is a white, bitter-tasting powder. Crystal meth has large, clear chunky crystals that look a bit like ice (hence the name).

In Southeast Asia and Australasia, the most predominant form of amphetamine used is crystalline methamphetamine (I'll go into more details about this at the end of the chapter). Methamphetamine must be metabolised into amphetamine in the body before it can be excreted, which is one explanation for why intoxication on methamphetamine lasts for longer than amphetamine sulphate.

I will use the term 'amphetamine' throughout the rest of this chapter to refer to amphetamine or methamphetamine, since most of the contents of this chapter apply to both, unless I am specifically talking about amphetamine sulphate, methamphetamine, or crystal meth, in which case I will use these terms.

---

* Although see later in the chapter: the term 'speed' might actually refer to methamphetamine these days. It certainly does in Australia.

Amphetamine can be consumed in a number of ways. It can be swallowed, snorted, injected, and crystal meth can also be 'smoked' in the same way as crack cocaine or heroin – heated until it turns to vapour then inhaled, rather than 'smoking' *per se.*

What are the short-term effects?

When amphetamine was initially investigated in the early 1930s, subjects reported increased feelings of wellbeing, confidence, alertness and energy. Amphetamine is a stimulant, so it has the classic stimulant effects of increasing heart rate and blood pressure, and of decreasing appetite.

How quickly a person begins to feel the effects of amphetamine will depend on the method of administration. If amphetamine is swallowed, it has to be absorbed through the stomach, and can take around half an hour to kick in. If snorted, intoxication will occur within minutes, and if smoked or injected, it will be almost instantaneous. Duration of intoxication is similarly variable, but it can last in the region of four to eight hours.

Amphetamine intoxication can induce feelings of confidence, wellbeing, alertness, motivation and focus. If snorted or injected, onset of intoxication can feel like a 'rush' of euphoria. People on amphetamine can appear more chatty and social, and they might also have an increased sex drive.

The combination of reducing tiredness and increasing energy has led some people to use amphetamine as a performance enhancer – there are reports of use among long-distance drivers (although the evidence is less than convincing about whether performance at tasks such as driving is actually improved, or the increased confidence caused by intoxication might lead a user to believe erroneously it has improved).

Amphetamine will increase a person's heart rate, blood pressure and body temperature, as all stimulants do. A person will experience a dry mouth and a lower appetite, and their pupils will dilate.

Many people report negative feelings as well as or instead of the positive ones described above. Amphetamine can increase anxiety and irritability, as well as causing restlessness and paranoia. There are many documented cases of amphetamine-induced psychosis, which can last days or weeks after taking the drug. Some surveys suggest these can occur in about 15 to 23 per cent of amphetamine users, and these symptoms can also be induced in experimental studies.

In almost all cases, the psychotic states will end after a person stops using amphetamine, although there is evidence that about one in five individuals who experience severe amphetamine-induced psychosis will go on to develop a prolonged psychotic disorder, potentially even schizophrenia.

If a person consumes too much amphetamine, they can experience extremely unpleasant symptoms, from difficulty breathing to fits or seizures and extreme agitation. Amphetamine overdose can lead to loss of consciousness, and in extreme circumstances to stroke, heart attack and death. It can also impact on the body's ability to regulate its own temperature, meaning a person is at risk of hyperthermia (overheating – the opposite of hypothermia).

Amphetamine can be dependence-inducing, and amphetamine withdrawal can cause tiredness, hunger, irritability and depression, as well as insomnia, mood swings and (as you might expect) craving for amphetamine. The comedown after taking amphetamine can last a couple of days (for individuals who do not use it regularly or are not dependent on the substance – in these cases withdrawal can be more severe).

What are the longer-term effects?

As for the risks from longer-term regular use of amphetamine over a number of years, this is harder to ascertain because studies are harder to do. Having said that, given how prevalent amphetamine prescribing was in the 1950s and 1960s, we do know a little about potential long-term risks from regular use – more so than for some other substances. As with all stimulants, a substance that increases heart rate and blood pressure can take its toll on the body, and chronic amphetamine use is linked with an increased risk of heart attack and stroke, particularly in those already at risk.

Similarly, amphetamine use has been linked to risk of irregular heartbeat. There's also evidence that long-term use of amphetamine increases the risk of glaucoma – a condition where pressure inside the eye damages the optic nerve. Case reports of amphetamine-induced glaucoma first appeared in medical journals in the 1960s. However, more recently a study found a higher correlation between cocaine use and risk of glaucoma than other illicit drugs, although amphetamine and cannabis use were also associated with an increased risk, so this risk is not necessarily specific to amphetamine.

There are further risks if a person is injecting amphetamine, including risks from repeated injecting and from poor needle hygiene. Injecting a drug also means that it enters the bloodstream – and the brain – very quickly, which can increase the potential for dependence to the substance to develop.

Heavy chronic amphetamine use has been found to be associated with increased levels of anhedonia – one of the symptoms of depression. Anhedonia is broadly defined as an inability to feel pleasure at things you have previously found pleasurable. As mentioned above, it has also been linked to risk of developing psychosis or psychotic disorder, as well as acute amphetamine-induced psychosis during intoxication. Regular amphetamine use is also linked to increased risk of symptoms of anxiety.

Brain-scan studies have repeatedly found differences in brain structure of populations defined as 'amphetamine abusers' – people who've used amphetamine frequently for a sustained period of time, compared to those who have not used amphetamine. In particular these differences are seen in grey matter, the volume of which is often reduced compared to healthy controls. Grey matter is located on the surface of the brain, and it's where the synapses – places where brain cells connect to each other – are located.

However, it's somewhat tricky to interpret what these differences between groups actually mean. These studies are almost always undertaken in heavy regular methamphetamine users. It's also extremely difficult to work out whether these differences are due to use of the drug, or whether pre-existing factors predict whether or not an individual is likely to start (and carry on) using methamphetamine. Perhaps the brain scans are picking up these differences, rather than those caused by the drug use.

In order to rule these potential alternative explanations out, we would need to take brain scans of individuals before they have ever used a drug, and then compare these to their brain after regular methamphetamine use. These studies haven't been conducted yet, because it's hard to predict who will go on to become a regular amphetamine user. Potentially, as brain scanning gets cheaper to conduct, studies might be conducted on a large enough scale that this becomes possible, but these would need to involve brain scans of many thousands of people.

Heavy amphetamine use, or amphetamine dependence, is associated with poor sleeping, poor nutrition, anorexia, and a prematurely aged appearance. Given some of the attributes of amphetamine, this makes some sense. Amphetamine is a stimulant, and as such can impact on sleep patterns. Stimulants are also appetite suppressants – which is why amphetamine has been marketed as a diet pill by many companies since it was first developed in the 1930s.

As such, people who are trying to reduce their weight might turn to it even now, when the risks of using it are better known. The suppression of appetite that amphetamine causes can easily lead to poor nutrition – not only are people eating less than perhaps they need to, but they may also turn to less healthy food when they do eat.

Myths and misconceptions

Speed can sober you up

I've heard people say that speed can sober up a person who has also been drinking alcohol, or that it can even be a way to get around a police breathalyser if a person is stopped for driving while drunk. There's absolutely no evidence that this is the case. Taking a stimulant while also drunk can mask the effect of both. But feelings can be deceiving – a person in this state certainly won't be able to drive, even if they feel like they might be.

It's also easier to overdose on either substance if their intoxication effects are masked by the presence of the other substance. Alcohol and amphetamine have been shown to interact together to increase heart rate and blood pressure beyond that caused by amphetamine alone. As such, the risk of heart attack or stroke is higher if an individual has also consumed alcohol, compared to when they've only consumed amphetamine.

 MYTH

Speed uses up a chunk of the finite number of beats your heart can do

All stimulants put a strain on your heart, and so using amphetamine regularly will increase a person's risk of cardio-vascular problems. But the heart doesn't have a 'finite number of beats' that means when it's overworked, you'll live shorter. If that was the case, people who spent their lives sitting on the sofa would live longer than those who increase their heart rates with regular exercise.

? PARTLY TRUE

Amphetamine rots your teeth

There are many case reports that suggest that regular use of amphetamine can increase the risk of poor dental hygiene. There's certainly evidence that regular use of the substance can lead to a dry mouth, and teeth grinding is a commonly experienced side-effect of intoxication. However, it's harder to say definitively whether it's the drug itself that is doing this, or whether other behaviours that the drug causes are leading to tooth damage.

For example, it's easy to see how poorer nutrition due to appetite suppression could impact on dental hygiene, and the impact amphetamine use has on an individual in terms of their sleep patterns and their general wellbeing could potentially lead to a person taking less care of oral cleanliness than they should. If the drug is consumed via the mouth, for instance by inhaling methamphetamine vapour, then this could also lead directly to tooth damage, and might increase the risk of some oral cancers as well.

However, there is some evidence that there might be something particularly risky about amphetamine, even compared to other drug use. A study conducted in 2008 in Melbourne, Australia, asked around 300 individuals who inject drugs about their substance use and their dental health. They found that amphetamine use was more commonly linked with poor dental health than heroin use, which might indicate that this is not entirely a myth.

? PARTLY TRUE

Does amphetamine have any medical uses?

Amphetamine was originally developed by the pharmaceutical industry, and has been prescribed as a medication since the 1930s. Some argue that it was the first psychoactive medication available. And it's been used to treat a number of conditions, from mild depression to hypochondria, Parkinsons to narcolepsy (a condition where an individual can fall asleep without warning or ability to prevent it happening). Amphetamine has been marketed as a diet pill and a pep pill, has been used during combat as a method of improving concentration, stamina and morale, and is prescribed today as a treatment for ADHD.

When amphetamine became arguably the first marketed anti-depressant medication, there was little evidence that it was effective. The man who patented it initially tested it upon himself (an alarmingly common practice), and noted the improvement on his mood. Studies were conducted to test this, and it was found that while amphetamine might relieve mild depression, it had properties that could exacerbate existing anxiety or psychosis-like traits.

Later, pharmaceutical companies mixed amphetamine with a barbiturate sedative to try and counter the anxiety-inducing aspects of the amphetamine, and prevent the drowsiness that came with barbiturates. Benzedrine inhalers, marketed to treat asthma, were available over the counter, and soon became popular both as a medication, and when people realised they could be cracked open and the amphetamine consumed via other methods.

As mentioned, amphetamine is currently prescribed to treat ADHD. It might seem counterintuitive to give a stimulant to an individual with hyperactivity problems, but evidence suggests that amphetamine can increase ability to concentrate, reduce instances of distraction, improve sustained attention and reduce impulsive behaviours – in populations with ADHD.

Amphetamine has long been used as a medication for promoting weight loss, due to the appetite suppressive nature of the substance. It became a particular issue in the USA in the late 1960s, where a regimen combining amphetamines with other substances to counteract some of their side-effects became known by the euphemistic term 'rainbow diet pills'.

It took deaths and an exposé of how easy it was to get prescriptions for these pills published in *Life* magazine in the USA for a change in legislation, which happened in 1970. Even so, certain amphetamine or amphetamine-based substances are still prescribed for obesity today.

What don't we know?

As is often the case with illicit substances, a white powder or a pill could contain anything. Substances might not be what they are sold as, and could be cut with all sorts of things. While researching this chapter, I found a number of references online that stated that 'speed' referred to methamphetamine. These seemed in most instances to come from Australia – where data from police seizures and other sources indicate that even substances sold as amphetamine are in almost all cases powdered methamphetamine.

Confusingly, in Australia certainly, and perhaps in other parts of the world, 'speed' seems to refer to both amphetamine sulphate and methamphetamine. Given that methamphetamine is more easily absorbed than amphetamine, and that intoxication on meth lasts longer, this may be increasing the risk of harm. Not to mention increasing the risk of confusion! It's worth pointing out that Australia has perhaps the most active researcher base investigating methamphetamine and amphetamine use across the world. As such, it's likely that monitoring evidence coming from Australia is more detailed, and it's also notable that (meth) amphetamine use is more prevalent in Australia and Southeast Asia than in other parts of the world.

When I spoke to researchers in Australia about this, they suggested that it may well be the case that methamphetamine is more widely used than amphetamine sulphate globally, and that 'speed' is quite likely to be methamphetamine rather than amphetamine sulphate in other parts of the world, too.

One final thing: amphetamine interacts dangerously with certain types of medication for depression and anxiety – specifically drugs known as MAOI inhibitors. It's extremely dangerous to take amphetamines if you are prescribed these.

CHAPTER 3

Benzodiazepines: Valium, Xanax, Rohypnol and more

ALPRAZOLAM (XANAX)

DIAZEPAM

What is it? Synthesised powder or pill, many different individual varieties.

Type of drug: Depressant – minor tranquiliser, to be more precise.

Popularity: Valium and Xanax are widely prescribed in the UK and USA for sleeping problems.

How consumed: Swallowed.

Timescale: Varies dependent on the type.

Some effects: Sedation of mind and muscle, impaired coordination, impaired ability to concentrate.

THE TERM BENZODIAZEPINE refers to a group of synthetic substances that have been used since the 1960s as a treatment for panic and anxiety. The first popular benzo was called Librium, but others that you may have heard of include diazepam (often known by the brand name Valium), alprazolam (Xanax), and rohypnol. There are numerous others as well, most of whose names end with –lam or –pam.

Benzodiazepines may be appealing because they are relatively easy to get compared to some other illicit drugs. It is possible to get prescriptions for some benzos in various countries around the world, although in many places such prescriptions are limited to the short-term, often no longer than four weeks at any time. Benzos might also be popular because they are a medication, so therefore could be perceived as safe compared to illicit substances made in bathtubs or DIY labs (though how true that is will be explored later).

What are the short-term effects?

Benzodiazepines are usually prescribed in a powder tablet, or occasionally a gel capsule form. If the substances are purchased from other sources, they can sometimes be found as a powder. As such, they are usually swallowed, but sometimes snorted. Some people will use gel capsules to create a liquid and inject benzos, but this is an extremely dangerous method of consumption. Although all benzos have broadly similar effects, each compound has a slightly different profile. For example, Xanax has a faster onset and a shorter intoxication period than Valium.

Benzos are known as 'minor tranquilisers' in the medical profession. This means a medicine to reduce symptoms of anxiety – one that has a minor sedative effect rather than a major effect, such as that required for the treatment of more severe mental health conditions like schizophrenia. They work by inducing sedation to mind and muscle. Some people describe experiencing a 'cosy sleepiness', or a 'calm chattiness' on low doses.

As expected, they can reduce feelings of anxiety, as well as feelings of tension and stress. Their physical sedation effect means that they can also lower coordination abilities, and impact on alertness and ability to concentrate. It's a very bad idea to drive, or operate other heavy machinery, when under the influence of benzodiazepines.

At higher doses, people can start slurring their speech, and experiencing more profound confusion. People are at increased risks of accidents because of the impact on coordination and concentration. The sedative effect could even lead to a loss of consciousness, or experiences of amnesia or blackouts (similar to those experienced at high levels of alcohol consumption).

Also similar to alcohol intoxication are the perhaps paradoxical reports of increased proneness to violent or aggressive behaviour from people intoxicated on benzos. While little is understood about why benzo intoxication might induce such behaviours, one theory is that benzodiazepines reduce inhibition, thus making a person more impulsive and likely to lash out, where they would otherwise resist the urge to do so.

If a person takes too high a dose and loses consciousness, they are at risk of choking on or inhaling their vomit. There is also a danger from the slowing and shallowing of breathing that benzodiazepines can produce, particularly in children, or individuals with pre-existing lung or breathing problems.

What are the longer-term effects?

If a person has been using benzos for a while, they will build up a tolerance to them, and require a larger dose to achieve the same effect. This is why, in the UK at least, prescriptions to benzodiazepines are broadly limited to two to four weeks at a time, rather than longer term. There is a risk of both a physical and psychological dependence to benzodiazepines after longer term and heavy use.

People who have used benzos in this way report a severe impact on their daily life from being mildly sedated at all times. Similarly, regular users report that anxiety levels can increase after a while of regular use, as well as feelings of panic, and sleep problems. People also report decreased energy levels. There have been anecdotal reports of an increased risk of dementia or memory problems in long-term users of benzos. However, there has been little research into this, and at present it is unclear whether these effects could reverse after a person stops taking the substance.

A person who has been regularly taking benzos can experience physical and psychological withdrawal when they stop taking them. Medical professionals advise seeking support if you want to quit benzos – ideally you will need to taper your dose down over a period of several months or possibly up to a year, depending on the level of use. GPs that I spoke to also suggested that psychological support such as cognitive behavioural therapy can be helpful, as individuals initially prescribed the substance for treating their anxiety may find that symptoms increase when they stop taking them.

Withdrawal symptoms also include an increased heart rate and blood pressure, the shakes, insomnia and sensitivity to light and sound. If a person tries to stop using benzodiazepines suddenly, they are at risk of more severe symptoms, such as seizures, which is why getting support is so strongly advised.

Myths and misconceptions

Benzos make highs from other drugs better

Benzodiazepines, when used recreationally rather than as prescribed, are very commonly used in conjunction with other drugs rather than by themselves (though this is not always the case). For example, survey data suggests that 30 to 50 per cent of individuals with alcohol dependence also use benzos. People report that benzos can enhance the intoxication experience of other depressants, such as alcohol or heroin. They can also reduce withdrawal effects from these substances, indeed benzodiazepines can sometimes be prescribed to help people going through alcohol withdrawal. Other people report using benzos to counter the effects of a stimulant they have consumed.

However, this sort of mixing can be really dangerous. Taking two depressants together (such as benzos and alcohol, or heroin) can increase the risk of an overdose, of blacking out and therefore the risk of choking, and of suffering ill effects from breathing being slowed. Conversely, mixing benzos with stimulants can mask the effects of both, meaning higher doses of both could be taken, putting extra strain on the heart and the liver, and increasing the risk of overdose, and tolerance building up.

There is also an increased likelihood of larger withdrawal effects, some of which could be potentially dangerous (as detailed earlier).

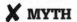 MYTH

Valerian tea is natural valium

Valerian is a herb that grows in Europe and Asia. The root has been used medicinally since ancient Greek and Roman times, and it's still marketed today as a herbal medicine to treat conditions such as insomnia, anxiety and restless leg syndrome. However, there's no known active ingredient in valerian root, and certainly not a benzodiazepine-like compound, although there's some inconclusive evidence that valerian root has an impact on a neurotransmitter called GABA, also implicated in the effects that benzos have.

But is there any evidence to support valerian tea having an effect on insomnia or anxiety? To date, there has been very little good-quality research conducted, and the evidence is pretty weak.

A systematic review of the literature on the link between valerian root and anxiety found only one study that had investigated this to a high standard, with only thirty-six participants. This study found no evidence that the effect of valerian was any different to a placebo, and weak evidence that diazepam, also tested, reduced anxiety symptoms to a greater degree than valerian root did. Similarly, a review investigating herbal medicine and insomnia found no evidence that valerian root is effective to treat this either.

 MYTH

Grapefruit juice can increase the high

There's something about grapefruit juice that interacts with a number of different medications. And included on that list are certain benzodiazepines, including diazepam, midazolam and triazolam. Grapefruit juice can result in slower metabolism of these substances, leading to a build-up of them in the blood. But rather than increasing the high, this is more likely to increase the risk of unwanted side-effects such as passing out or loss of coordination.

Other medications can also interact with benzodiazepines in this way, including antihistamines and some other medications that treat depression.

? PARTLY TRUE

Do benzos have medical uses?

Benzodiazepines were initially discovered in the mid-1950s, and were investigated as a potential medication to treat anxiety after animal studies found that Librium, the first to be synthesised, made mice relaxed and drowsy. At the time, barbiturates were used to treat anxiety, but these had a high risk of negatively impacting on a person's ability to breathe properly. Librium, and then a few years later Valium, immediately became extremely popular, particularly in the USA. By the 1970s they were topping 'most prescribed medication' lists, but by the 1980s it was becoming more obvious that there were risks of dependence from long-term prescriptions.

While these risks are still very real, benzodiazepines are still prescribed across the world today, most commonly as a short-term treatment for conditions such as panic disorder, generalised anxiety disorder or insomnia. Benzodiazepines can also be used in conditions where people have seizures, as the sedation effect of the compound can quell these – for example, people with epilepsy who have prolonged seizures, and people experiencing alcohol withdrawal, where it can ease agitation and trembles that can occur.

Benzos are sometimes prescribed for pre-surgery anxiety, and can also be used in a medical setting to reduce panic in individuals having a bad reaction to intoxication on a hallucinogen.

What don't we know?

There's some evidence that there might be a risk to the foetus if benzos are used during pregnancy. There is a small increase in the risk of the baby being born with a cleft palate, although the overall risk is low, and the evidence to date suggesting a causal link is not strong.

Most of this research has been conducted on individuals who were prescribed benzodiazepines during pregnancy, and who therefore were likely to be experiencing conditions such as anxiety or epilepsy, which could also increase the risk of complications during pregnancy. Similarly, many of the women in these studies were taking other medication as well, so pinpointing the effect to benzodiazepines specifically is challenging.

There are anecdotal reports of babies being born with what is referred to as 'floppy infant syndrome' if benzos are used very close to birth. Symptoms of this can include poor muscle tone in the infant, sedation, impaired metabolic responses to experiencing coldness, or reluctance to suckle. These symptoms have been found to last somewhere between a few hours up to some months after the baby was born.

However, there is little evidence that these symptoms are associated with longer-term problems in the child, and whether the use of benzodiazepines during pregnancy is a significant risk that outweighs the potential benefits they might have is not clear.

Outside of benzodiazepine prescription, problematic patterns of benzo use have been found in survey studies to be linked to socio-economic factors such as being in receipt of government benefits, being homeless, and having previously been incarcerated. This is quite a complicated finding to unpick – is it that people with these backgrounds or experiences are more likely to be drawn to using benzodiazepines? Or does regular consumption of a sedating substance like benzos make holding down a job harder, or maintaining social networks more of a challenge?

In all likelihood it is a complex relationship operating in both directions, and it's also important to remember that most people using benzodiazepines will also use other substances, particularly alcohol and heroin, and that the use of benzos along with these substances often predicts more problematic and dangerous use, and poorer outcomes, than using those substances without using benzos as well. The majority of people who use benzos but do not use other substances tend to do so after initially being prescribed them, perhaps highlighting how difficult it is to stop taking benzos once you've started.

When I was growing up, the benzodiazepine that I had heard of, because of many media reports, was temazepam. Data collected in 1987 suggested that it was the prescription drug most commonly used illicitly across the UK. It was particularly used among people who injected drugs, according to a study in 1994, and was implicated in a rise in drug-related deaths in the early 1990s in Scotland. Because of these harms,* temazepam is no longer available on the NHS, and if pharmacies stock it for private prescriptions, they have to follow strict restrictions, for instance storing it in safe custody on their premises. Prescriptions have to go through a special controlled-drug prescription form.

Why was temazepam so problematic during this period? It is possibly because of its profile compared to other benzodiazepines, such as speed of onset and duration of effect. But it may also be more prosaically due to availability. Temazepam was around, so it was used. Also, it was possible to get temazepam as a gel, meaning it could be injected. Since the change in legislation, it is only available as a solid tablet, minimising this possibility.

Today, Xanax (the brand name, the substance is alprazolam) is getting a lot of media attention in the UK. Xanax is a prescription medication (although not available on the NHS, so not – or certainly only very rarely – prescribed in the UK), but illicit Xanax may have been made outside of a pharmaceutical company.

If this is the case, then the quality and dosage contained within any one tablet is immediately less easy to predict – it's unlikely that people making their own Xanax will be able to make it to the same standard as a pharmaceutical company, even if they wanted to. And that's assuming it really is Xanax in the first place – if a person buys an illicit substance over the internet, there is no guarantee that they will receive what they have ordered.

Headlines in the UK have claimed that young people are buying 'fake' Xanax over the internet, and experiencing severe negative consequences, including overdose and death. There have been cases where the 'Xanax' was actually nothing of the sort,

---

* And perhaps the media attention, too.

sometimes instead containing opioids, or other psychoactive substances.

In Wales there is a postal-based service that will test samples of drugs mailed to it, called WEDINOS. In their 2017–2018 annual report, they detailed having received an increase in benzodiazepines being submitted to the service (behind more commonly sent substances like cocaine and MDMA). However, they also found that a large proportion of the 'benzodiazepine' samples submitted to them in reality contained either a different benzo to the one the sender believed was present, or a different substance entirely (some samples submitted as Xanax were actually caffeine tablets, for example).

Taking a substance without knowing what is in it can greatly increase the risk of harm.

Focus on: Comedowns

Why do people feel rubbish for a day (or two) after taking a substance? From alcohol to amphetamine, MDMA to ketamine, stimulants and depressants can lead to a comedown, or hangover, after the intoxication has ended.

What symptoms do people experience?

Comedowns can be physical and emotional in nature. A pounding head and nausea are common hangover symptoms. People can feel achy and exhausted after taking a substance, their stomach might be upset, or they might feel ravenously hungry. And that's before we get onto the emotional side of a comedown.

People can feel really down, shedding a tear at the most unexpected thing, or feel quite emotionally 'flat'. Symptoms of anxiety are also a feature of some comedowns, and some people feel irritable as well.

What causes a comedown?

It's surprisingly hard to research the after-effects of taking a substance. This is true for regulated drugs like alcohol, and even more so for illicit substances. While you can bring people into a lab and give them a substance and see what happens, it's more challenging to keep them there for a day or two to find out what happens afterwards!

Even so, we understand a bit about what causes people to feel ropey following an evening of excess.

Headaches are likely to be caused by dehydration – not only do some drugs impact how the body absorbs water, and how a person then expels it afterwards, but they also impact on judgment and might lead a person to be less likely to look after themselves while intoxicated.

Exhaustion is a common comedown symptom, and this is very probably because drugs can impact on the amount and quality of sleep a person has. Stimulants clearly interfere with sleep, but even drugs like alcohol will impact on the quality of sleep you have. Substances will also play a role in the type of things you get up to while intoxicated. And this can affect the comedown – surprisingly enough, people who are leaping around in a club until 5 a.m. will feel worse the next day than people who spent the evening at home on the sofa.

Psychoactive substances also impact neurotransmitters in the brain. MDMA, for example, is thought to increase the levels of serotonin in the brain. And what goes up must come down – there's some suggestion that serotonin levels will fall below their baseline levels in the day or two following MDMA use, before they return to normal.

Another potential reason people might feel rough after taking drugs is because the body might react to them, or adulterants they might contain, as something dangerous to it – a poison –

and try and get rid of it. This might explain stomach problems, vomiting and diarrhoea. And, of course, individual differences between people, in terms of their genetics, their metabolism, their liver function, hormone levels, and all sorts of things, will impact on their ability to bounce back after intoxication.

Can a comedown be avoided?

A comedown can easily be avoided – by not taking a substance the night before. For people who do take a substance, some of the symptoms can be mitigated. Headaches can be minimised by drinking water, or even better isotonic drinks to replace any electrolytes you might have sweated out.

Allowing yourself time to recover will help deal with the exhaustion you might feel – and if you are feeling physical symptoms such as tremors or impaired vision, it is dangerous to consider driving or operating heavy machinery, even if you wanted to.

CHAPTER 4

Caffeine

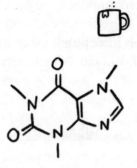

What is it? Compound found in various plants, can also be
synthesised.
Type of drug: Stimulant.
Popularity: Globally popular, and globally legal.
How consumed: Usually drunk, although can be taken as a
supplement in powder form.
Timescale: Peak effects around 45 minutes after consumption.
Some effects: Small increase in alertness, concentration,
reduction in drowsiness, increase in blood pressure.

YES, CAFFEINE IS a drug. Even if you've avoided every single other
substance in this book, I'd be willing to bet that almost everyone,
barring people with severe allergies or intolerances, has consumed
a product containing caffeine at some point in their lives. Caffeine,
particularly in beverages, is consumed around the globe, be it in
colas, coffee, tea, or maté – the national drink of Paraguay,
Uruguay and Argentina.

Most drinks and food products containing caffeine are not regulated – cans of cola are consumed by children worldwide, even if they turn their noses up at more 'grown-up' cups of tea (as I used to when I was young, eventually filling the teacup with sugar in an attempt to make it more palatable). But caffeine is a drug – a methylated xanthine to be precise – it has a stimulant effect, there's some suggestion it can be dependence forming for some people (possibly more people than you might think, possibly even you reading this), and it most certainly has withdrawal symptoms.

What is it?

As you probably already know, caffeine is found in coffee and tea, two of the most popular hot drinks across the world. And many people are aware that caffeine is also found in chocolate, albeit at much lower levels. There is more caffeine in dark chocolate compared to milk, and the amount is broadly similar to the higher end of levels found in decaf tea and coffee – some caffeine remains in these despite their name.

Caffeine occurs naturally in approximately sixty plant species, including tea leaves and coffee beans; guarana berries, used to make a number of energy snacks and drinks; kola nuts, which were once used to make cola drinks (although this is less common now), and yerba maté.

I had never heard of maté until I went to Uruguay a few years ago. Montevideo was an incredible city and I really fell in love with it while I was there, but I was fascinated with a pastime that everyone, from groups of teens on the beach to retired couples taking the air, seemed to be partaking of. Almost every person we passed was carrying with them what looked to be a wooden bowl-like vessel, with a metal straw sticking out of the top.

If you think a nice pot of tea is an English obsession, this took it to the next level. As we walked along the beach path, every bench we passed was occupied by people enjoying the view and their mysterious drink.

Luckily, I was travelling with a Syrian friend who was able to tell me all about maté – by coincidence Syria is the largest importer of the drink. It's a hot infusion made in a way much like tea, by steeping dried yerba maté leaves in near-boiling water. The calabash gourd keeps the water warm, and the metal straw has a second role acting as a sieve to keep the large pieces of plant out of your mouth while you drink. The taste isn't a million miles away from a classic English breakfast tea either, probably due to the tannins contained by both. It's perhaps a little more 'woody', certainly if there are stems included as well as leaves in the preparation.

Maté has also made it to Europe – in Germany, Club Mate is a fizzy drink made of maté, and is somewhat similar to cola, although containing lower sugar levels and fewer calories.

As well as products that naturally contain caffeine, it's possible to manufacture caffeine as a powder, which can then be added as a supplement to drinks and food. For example, energy drinks such as Red Bull, Monster and the like contain caffeine that is added rather than naturally contained. And it's in some drinks you might not expect. A can of Sunkist orange contains 41mg of caffeine – that's higher than a can of Coca-Cola, which contains 34mg. Cola drinks are interesting, in that they were initially made using kola nuts, but these days a cola is more likely to contain synthetic caffeine and not the kola nut.

What's considered a 'dose' of caffeine?

A few years ago, I read a great book called *Caffeinated* by Murray Carpenter. In it, he suggests that around 75mg of caffeine is a 'standard caffeine dose', or Scad as he calls it. This is conceptually similar to a unit of alcohol, and different caffeine-containing products contain different amounts.

For example, a Scad is roughly equal to a 60ml espresso, or a small cup of filter coffee. Black tea contains slightly less caffeine, about 50mg per mug. A can of an energy drink is roughly the same as an espresso, one Scad. Two cans of cola are equivalent to a Scad, or a pint of Diet Coke. A 50g bar of plain chocolate contains on average 25mg of caffeine – so you'd have to eat 150g to get an espresso kick. And as we discussed earlier, there's even less in milk chocolate – you'd need 500g to get a Scad's worth of caffeine.

Having said all that, those are averages, and given how we make hot beverages in particular, mixing grounds, leaves or an instant mix with water, how long we leave the bag in or how long we let a cafetière steep will all impact on how much caffeine ends up in your drink. Not only that but the level of caffeine in an individual coffee bean or tea leaf is not consistent, being affected by natural growing conditions and the variety of bean. But surely it can't be *that* varied, right? You'd be surprised.

In 2014, a group of researchers went to a variety of cafés across Glasgow in Scotland, Parma in Italy, and Pamplona in Spain, on four separate occasions. At each café they visited, they ordered an espresso, and then measured the caffeine it contained. What they found was extremely interesting.

Firstly, espressos in Scotland were quite inconsistent in volume. One café was serving tiny espressos at 15ml a pop. In another an order of an espresso would give you 52ml of coffee. In Italy there was more consistency, with an espresso being between 15 and 27ml. Espressos in Spain were bigger and ranged between 50 and 83ml.

The levels of caffeine within these drinks were surprisingly inconsistent, both between shops and even on different visits to the same shop. In Glasgow the mean caffeine per drink ranged from 72mg all the way up to 212mg – and these variations were not totally explained by the drink size. In Italy the caffeine in an espresso ranged between 73 and 135mg, and in Spain between 97 and 127mg. So you might think that your usual coffee will always contain the same amount of caffeine, but this is not necessarily the case. I've certainly experienced some days where no matter how much coffee I drink it doesn't seem to have an effect, while on other days I'll feel jittery and uncomfortable after one cup. And this may well be why.

What are the short-term effects?

After you eat or drink a product containing caffeine, there's a bit of a delay before any onset of intoxication, although some studies have found an impact of caffeine on reaction-time tasks within minutes of consuming it. Caffeine levels will ramp up over time and by around 45 minutes after consumption they will be at peak levels. The effect of caffeine will then usually last around three to four hours before wearing off.

Caffeine is a mild stimulant, and as such, it can have a small effect on a person's alertness, their concentration, wakefulness, and some studies have suggested it can improve reaction times. Caffeine can also reduce feelings of drowsiness (though this may only be in individuals habituated to caffeine, bringing them out of withdrawal), and some studies have suggested it can improve concentration and accuracy in individuals who are sleep-deprived, although only up to a certain point (nothing is a substitute for adequate sleep, particularly if you need to do something like operate machinery or drive a car).

Caffeine consumption seems to cause a short spike in blood pressure. This may be happening via vasoconstriction – the narrow-ing of blood vessels. This vasoconstriction is particularly pronounced in the brain, and may be why people get headaches when they stop drinking coffee after doing so regularly. Caffeine can also increase feelings of anxiety, and impact on motor functioning.

Caffeine is a fairly common supplement in sporting environments. Evidence suggests it can improve sprinting speed, cycling ability, and aid with endurance activities.

It's commonly known that caffeine is a diuretic – a substance that will make a person urinate more. This is true, although this is not really the case in the doses that most people consume it in. As an example, an individual would need to drink two or three coffees in very quick succession, or somewhere between five and eight cups of tea, in order to experience this (and let's be honest, that amount of liquid is going to make you need the loo anyway!).

It is possible to consume too much caffeine, and the effects of doing so can be unpleasant. Caffeine toxicity can cause dizziness, anxiety, the shakes or a jittery feeling, and heart palpitations. At extremely high levels, caffeine can be fatal. It would be difficult to consume this amount of caffeine through drinks, such as 200 cups of tea or 50 coffees. There have been a number of media articles implicating energy drinks in individual fatalities. Even with very high-caffeine energy drinks, it would be exceedingly hard to drink the amount of liquid that would contain that level of caffeine.

However, other medications or foods or supplements also contain caffeine, so it is not impossible that caffeine was implicated in these deaths. It may also be the case that the individuals also had other underlying health problems that made them more vulnerable to the effects of caffeine, or potentially that other substances were involved as well – for example, mixing alcohol and energy drinks can increase the risk of harm.

More recently, it has become easier to buy powdered caffeine, and caffeine pills. Caffeine is also often found in pills that claim to aid dieting, such as ketone pills. It is clearly much easier to overdose on caffeine via these methods, where the caffeine can be consumed in a more concentrated form, without copious amounts of liquid alongside it.

Given caffeine is a mild stimulant and can reduce feelings of drowsiness, it can also cause insomnia in some people. If you drink a cup of coffee to wake yourself up at 8 p.m., you might still be feeling the stimulating effects at midnight. I've always had insomnia, and so I avoid caffeine after around 4 p.m., although I'm aware that there could well be some level of psychosomatic input here – if I'm worried I won't be able to sleep, or if I'm feeling overtired, my insomnia gets worse, so it's perfectly possible that if I have a late cup of tea I'm already expecting to sleep badly, and it becomes somewhat of a self-fulfilling prophecy. Annoying!

Caffeine intoxication might give you a very small increased risk of a heart attack, as is the case with a number of other stimulants. Studies have reliably shown that caffeine will increase a person's blood pressure, and this is an effect that does not seem to disappear with tolerance to caffeine. However, this is extremely unlikely unless you have other underlying health problems, and even then it is very rare.

What are the longer-term effects?

Caffeine is a stimulant, and it's a stimulant that a lot of people take very regularly, possibly multiple times every day for many decades of their lives. What is it doing to us? Some observational studies have found a link between caffeine use and risk of cardiovascular disease – the narrowing or blocking of blood vessels that can lead to heart attacks, angina, or stroke.

However, the pattern of results found is quite unusual. Researchers found that high levels of caffeine increase the risk for the disease, but not in everyone – some studies suggest this is only in individuals under fifty-five, some find no such effect, and others find that moderate amounts of caffeine might be protective.

In 2014, a systematic review of all the studies that looked at the link between coffee and cardiovascular disease was published.

These results suggested a small protective effect of three to five coffees a day, and no great increase of risk for heavier coffee consumption (more on this study later).

We do know that habitual caffeine consumption can lead to caffeine withdrawal when a person stops consuming it. The symptoms of caffeine withdrawal might be familiar to anyone who's tried to cut down. They can include headaches, lethargy, an inability to concentrate, depression, irritability, and aches and pains including stomach and joint pain. Sometimes it's only when you stop that you realise the effect that something is having on you! And these symptoms are fairly common. Around half of people who drink two or three coffees per day, who go into withdrawal, will experience headaches.

If you are keen to quit caffeine, it's worth tapering down your dose if you want to avoid these symptoms – otherwise they should pass within a few days of stopping.

Myths and misconceptions

For such a commonly used substance, there are a load of myths and misconceptions about caffeine. Here are some of my favourites.

There's more caffeine in tea than coffee

I think the root of this misconception is largely well understood by people now, due in no small part to the British TV programme *QI*, where it's been extensively debunked. It is true that by dry weight, tea leaves contain more caffeine than coffee beans. But once you've brewed your tea or percolated your coffee (and bearing in mind the large variation in caffeine levels detailed above), in the resulting drink there will on average be substantially more caffeine in a mug of coffee than a mug of tea.

 MYTH

Green tea has no caffeine

This one really depends on your brewing technique. Green and black tea leaves on average contain similar amounts of caffeine, so again it comes down to personal preference – the amount of caffeine that makes it into your cuppa will be dependent on how long you steep it for, how much you stir the pot, how hot you have the water when you add it to the leaves, and such like. But green tea isn't a caffeine-free alternative to builder's tea.

 MYTH

It's impossible to have too much caffeine

I heard this myth first-hand, at an event encouraging women to get into cycling, spoken by a man claiming to be a sports scientist. As has been detailed extensively above, this is very much not the case. Caffeine overdose is unpleasant, it won't make riding a bike easier (quite the opposite), and too much caffeine can be fatal, particularly if consumed as a supplement rather than in a beverage, where consuming higher quantities is easier as the caffeine is far more concentrated.

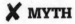 **MYTH**

Caffeine doesn't have any effect unless you're already using it

This is only partly a myth. All the physiological effects of caffeine will occur whether you've used it before or not. And in fact, due to tolerance, they might even have a stronger effect in people unaccustomed to caffeine. But there's also a growing body of evidence that suggests that a lot of the seemingly cognitive-enhancing effects of coffee – the improvement in alertness and concentration, maybe even reaction time – might actually be a reversal of the impairment of caffeine withdrawal.

A study led by a former colleague of mine in Bristol, Professor Peter Rogers, investigated the impact of caffeine on regular users who had been asked to abstain overnight before the study, and people who rarely or never consume it. Individuals came to the lab in the morning, around 10.30 a.m. They were given some baseline tasks to do, then given either caffeine or a placebo at around 11.15 a.m., and again at 12.45 p.m. The experiment involved two further testing sessions, at 1.45 p.m. and 3.30 p.m.

Rogers and his colleagues found that of the 379 participants recruited into this fairly epic study, those who reported hardly ever or never consuming caffeine got no benefit on various cognitive tasks from consuming caffeine, while the abstinent coffee-drinkers showed improvement when given caffeine compared to those who were given placebo, but only up to the level that the non-coffee drinkers were already operating at, whether they had placebo or caffeine.

Further analysis of data from the same experiment found that caffeine appeared to decrease sleepiness in those who did not normally consume it, even after just one dose. However, there was no evidence that caffeine improved performance on reaction-time or memory tasks for people who didn't usually consume caffeine. And conversely, for people used to higher levels of caffeine but in the placebo condition, their performance was markedly worse, particularly later in the afternoon.*

? PARTLY TRUE

---

* As a minor aside, I know these results quite well, because Peter was interviewed by a German TV company about this research. As part of it, the company wanted to 're-enact' the study so they could film it. I was a research assistant loitering around the department the day they were filming, and I got roped in to play the part of a high-caffeine consumer, beginning the day being sluggish, but after receiving my dose of caffeine perking right up! I really tested my acting chops that day.

Decaffeinated coffee and tea still contain caffeine

This isn't a myth. It is not possible to create coffee or tea that doesn't contain any caffeine. Decaf beverages are usually made by stripping the caffeine out of the tea leaves or coffee beans, and this removes most but not all of the caffeine. This is normally done with solvents such as methylene chloride or ethyl acetate, which are themselves then removed, or using carbon dioxide. There is a third possible process called the water process (or Swiss water process, after the company that performs it), which uses water and a separate batch of green coffee beans with caffeine removed to draw the caffeine out of the beans. This method is not possible for tea.

It's generally the case that decaffeinated drinks contain an order-of-magnitude lower dose of caffeine than their caffeinated relative (at least ten to twenty times less caffeine). Some studies where low doses of caffeine have been administered suggest that a psychoactive effect can still be felt even at these levels, so if you want to eliminate caffeine completely from your life, decaffeinated teas and coffees might need to go as well.

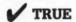 **TRUE**

Does caffeine have any medical uses?

As we discussed earlier, there is now some evidence that a small amount of caffeine per day could be protective against cardio-vascular disease. That said, it's important to remember that this finding came from observational studies – looking at what people choose to do. It might be the case that people who drink that amount of coffee are different from people who don't, in lots of other ways (amount of exercise, amount of alcohol, likelihood to smoke . . . it could be any number of things) that could also impact on cardiovascular health.

But there are some ways in which caffeine can be beneficial. You might notice when you take a powdered cold and flu medication, or some brands of ibuprofen or paracetamol, that these pills also contain caffeine. Usually it's around 100mg, so a fairly decent whack of caffeine. Studies have found that the addition of caffeine to these pain medications can make them a small amount more effective, although the evidence isn't strong.

Some researchers believe that the addition of caffeine to these medications helps prevent the caffeine-withdrawal headaches that can occur if the symptoms of their cold or flu are making a person less likely to drink their usual tea or coffee. Similarly, there's some evidence that pain after an operation can be worse if a person is unable to have their regular caffeine intake, so supplements are often given alongside other pain medication in this circumstance as well.

Caffeine citrate, a citric acid salt of caffeine, is on the World Health Organisation's list of essential medicines. It is used to treat or prevent infant breathing disorders, particularly in premature babies.

Caffeine has also been implicated in a number of other diseases, including Parkinson's. Findings – again observational – have suggested that consuming caffeine could be protective against Parkinson's (interestingly these same studies were able to compare those who consumed caffeinated versus decaffeinated coffee, and decaf didn't seem to show this protective effect). Strangely, this effect is seen only in men, not women. If caffeine can protect against Parkinson's, then it could be extremely important, as there is currently no cure for the disease. As yet, randomised controlled trials have not found anything conclusive regarding caffeine.

However, in early 2018, Japanese researchers published some findings that suggest caffeine might have another use. They assessed the blood levels of caffeine in people with and without

Parkinson's, and found a difference between the groups, even though they had consumed the same amount of caffeine. The authors suggested that perhaps blood caffeine levels could provide an early indication of whether an individual has Parkinson's or not – a diagnostic test for the disease.

It's still early days, as it is not yet clear whether blood caffeine levels are also different in other neurological conditions, or whether this could distinguish Parkinson's from these as well. And it's also not clear why this difference in blood caffeine level was seen. As is so often the case, further research is needed.

What about cancer? Everything either causes or cures cancer, right? Some things even seem to do both. Well, the good news is that in 2016 the International Agency for Research on Cancer reviewed thousands of studies and concluded that there's no strong evidence that coffee increases your chance of cancer. And some studies have gone further and suggested that coffee might perhaps reduce the risk of some cancers, specifically liver cancer and womb cancer. The studies show that these types of cancer are less common in people who drink coffee – but like a number of the other studies we've discussed, they can't really tell us anything about causation.

It is also worth noting that the IARC, mentioned above, have also concluded that very hot drinks, hotter than 65°C, 'probably cause cancer', specifically oesophageal cancer. This is a potential cause for concern for people in Middle Eastern countries and South America – maté is often consumed at this temperature, but coffee and most other teas are usually drunk when they are cooler than 65°C.

CHAPTER 5

Cannabis

What is it? A plant; the psychoactive cannabinoids (there are hundreds) are mostly found in the leaves and buds of the plant.

Type of drug: Belongs in its own category really.

Popularity: Changing – the legality of cannabis is changing across the world, for both medical and recreational use.

How consumed: Usually smoked, can be vaped or eaten.

Timescale: Peaks around half an hour after smoking, duration of 2 to 4 hours.

Some effects: Mellow and giggly or anxious and paranoid, increase in heart rate, muscle relaxation, increase in hunger.

CANNABIS, ALSO KNOWN as marijuana, herb, weed, pot, mary jane and myriad other colloquialisms, is a plant found indigenously in Central Asia and India, and also grown in the USA and Canada, among other places. It has uses aside from as a psychoactive substance – hemp is a strain of cannabis plant grown to produce fibres, which are used for all sorts of things from clothes to paper, plastics to animal feed.

Cannabis the drug refers to the resin or flowering buds of the plant, where the psychoactive compounds can be found. The drug is usually consumed by smoking these parts, which can be prepared in a variety of ways. These can then be smoked (sometimes with, sometimes without tobacco), eaten (often baked into biscuits or cakes), or more recently, vaped (using a heat-not-burn device that evaporates the cannabinoids from the plant material).

There are two strains of cannabis – indica and sativa.* Many people believe that these different variants of cannabis induce different intoxication effects. However, there's no evidence to back this up – rather the intoxication effects from cannabis of any kind will depend on the active compounds in the plant.

Cannabis's active compounds are called, rather originally, cannabinoids.† The one you might have heard of is delta-9-tetrahydrocannabinol, or THC. This is often called 'the active ingredient' in cannabis, but actually there are over 144 known cannabinoids, and in all likelihood there may be even more. THC is the compound that has been most rigorously researched, but more recently another cannabinoid called cannabidiol, known as CBD, has sparked interest in researchers. More on that later.

Cannabinoids interact with the endocannabinoid system in the brain. That's right, we actually have cannabinoid-like compounds that occur naturally in our brains and bodies. The neurotransmitter anandamide is an endocannabinoid found in

---

* There are also a *lot* of hybrids that are crossbreeds of indica and sativa strains, in fact most cannabis is probably a hybrid to a greater or lesser extent.

† As well as cannabinoids found in the cannabis plant, it's also possible to make synthetic cannabinoids that have related but different properties to the cannabinoids found in cannabis. Spice is one example of this, and is detailed in a separate chapter.

our brains. There are a couple of types of cannabinoid receptors – known, again rather originally, as CB1 and CB2.

CB1 receptors are mainly in the brain (though some are found elsewhere in the body), but CB2 receptors are found all over the body. Our endocannabinoid system is involved with processes such as mood, appetite, memory and pain perception. THC is what's called a 'partial agonist' of CB1 and CB2 receptors. This means it partially activates the receptors that control the flow of neurotransmitters across the gaps between neurons (the other way a compound can act on a receptor is as an 'antagonist', which, as it sounds, has the opposite effect).

Cannabis is the most widely used illicit drug* in the UK, and indeed most of the Western world. Despite the common perception that cannabis might be linked to poor mental health and educational outcomes, it is popular in part because it's seen as less harmful than some other illicit drugs, and not necessarily that different to smoking cigarettes. But does the evidence back up this belief?

What are the short-term effects?

Cannabis has an intoxication effect that peaks around fifteen to thirty minutes after smoking, and can last for two to four hours. If you eat cannabis it takes longer before you start to feel high, but intoxication can then last even longer. As you might expect, because of this lag it's hard to judge how much to consume if

---

* Is cannabis still an illicit drug? At the time of writing this, cannabis is now legal in Canada at a Federal level. It's legal in Uruguay. At state level it is legal in 11 USA states, and decriminalised in 8 more. It's legal for medical use only in a further 22 states. The UK has just announced that medications containing THC will be able to be prescribed by certified doctors from 1 November 2018. In all likelihood this will have changed again between this book going to print and you reading it. Sorry about that, I don't make the rules (or policy!)

you eat it, meaning it's far easier to misjudge the dose and take too much, leading to a pretty unpleasant experience that you can do very little about, other than wait for it to be over.

People report feeling giggly, mellow and sleepy while high. But cannabis intoxication can also induce psychotic-like feelings, paranoia, anxiety, occasionally even hallucinations. These almost always dissipate when a person is no longer intoxicated.

Physically, cannabis intoxication is associated with an increase in heart rate, a dry mouth, red eyes, and muscle relaxation. Because of the effect on blood pressure and the heart, there's a small increased risk of heart attack for about an hour after smoking, roughly equivalent to the increase in risk caused by vigorous exercise, or having sex.

If you take too much cannabis you can feel sick, find it difficult to move or speak, and find it hard to control your limbs. Cannabis can also lead to a drop in blood pressure, and a feeling of light-headedness, faintness, and nausea – the 'whitey', as it's known. It's also common to feel really hungry while high – the munchies. This is because our feelings of hunger are controlled by endocannabinoids, so consuming cannabis messes with them and induces hunger.

What are the longer-term effects?

It is much more difficult to conduct research to understand the longer-term effects of cannabis, or any substance for that matter. Double-blind randomised controlled trials (RCTs) are possible when looking at short-term intoxication effects, and indeed such studies have been done.

The first of these was published by Yale University psychiatrist and researcher Professor D'Souza and his colleagues in 2004. They ran a small but well-designed study on twenty-two healthy individuals in Connecticut, USA. Each participant came into the lab three times for an injection. On one occasion they got a placebo – an injection of ethanol (alcohol), but at a low enough level not to elicit any psychoactive effects. On the other two occasions the ethanol injection contained additional THC, at two different concentrations.

The participants didn't know which they were getting, and neither did the experimenter. This is what's known as a 'double blind' experiment, and it helps to eliminate reporting bias – if the participant is aware they are getting THC, they might have an expectation of how that would make them feel, which could skew the results. And if the experimenter knows, they might accidentally behave differently in the different conditions – ask leading questions or that sort of thing. Double-blind experiments are something to strive for where they are possible.

The researchers then took a load of measures from the participants, and found that those who'd been given THC at either level reported feeling higher levels of what are known as the positive symptoms of psychosis. These are things like paranoia, loss of insight, and 'grandiosity'. The researchers even recorded some of the things the participants said after they had taken part in the study. 'I felt as if my mind was nude', 'I thought you could read my mind, that's why I didn't answer', 'My thoughts were fragmented, the past, present and the future seemed to be happening at once', even 'I thought I was God'.

These are called positive symptoms because they are additional things and feelings happening to a person that shouldn't be. The participants in the study also reported negative symptoms of psychosis while intoxicated with THC. These, conversely, are the absence of things that a person should be experiencing, and can include a flattening of emotions, poor rapport with the experimenter, seeming distracted, that sort of thing. The ethanol 'placebo' condition didn't affect reporting of either the positive or the negative symptoms.

Now this might all sound quite lurid and worrying, but it was very short-lived. Individuals in the study stopped experiencing these symptoms within around three hours of being injected. In other words, these were intoxication effects that went away as soon as a participant was no longer high.

If we want to understand the longer-term impact of regular cannabis use, we have to rely on observing what people choose to do, while accounting for the other differences that might exist between people who choose to use cannabis, and people who choose not to. And this is assuming that people tell the truth when they are asked about their substance use in the first place.

It's possible that smoking cannabis will confer similar physical health risks to smoking tobacco. The process of burning the cannabis is likely to release carcinogens, and the common practice of smoking cannabis mixed with tobacco means the risks associated with smoking such as lung, throat and mouth cancers are likely to apply for cannabis, too.

Research has been somewhat inconclusive as to the risk of lung cancer from cannabis use. A paper using data from the International Lung Cancer Consortium published in 2015 found little evidence for a link between cannabis smoking and lung cancer in individuals who had never used tobacco, though they also state that harm from long-term heavy consumption cannot be ruled out by their findings.

There's been some research that has suggested a link between cannabis use and risk of heart disease and stroke, but at present the evidence is not strong. Of course, lack of evidence doesn't necessarily mean the risk isn't there, just that we can't be sure.

Heavy cannabis use has been implicated in an increased risk for some mental health problems, in particular psychotic disorders such as schizophrenia. Since cannabis use can induce psychotic experiences while a person is intoxicated, this is perhaps not surprising (although other risk factors for psychosis don't necessarily induce acute psychotic symptoms).

There's pretty consistent evidence from observational studies that very heavy cannabis use during teenage years predicts a small, but important, increase in risk for schizophrenia later. However, given how common cannabis use is, and how rare schizophrenia is, cannabis cannot be either necessary or sufficient to cause schizophrenia. It may be the case that cannabis is one risk factor among many, and for certain people who have a family history of schizophrenia for example, or other risk factors for the disorder, it could lead to problems, while for most people it won't. This is what I have spent many years researching – and I don't think we have a definitive answer yet.

The trouble is, at the moment there isn't a good way of identifying who's likely to be at higher risk. Other risk factors for psychosis include family history of similar mental health problems, living in an urban environment, being a migrant, childhood adversity, and several others. Individuals who fit in these categories may be particularly at risk from cannabis use, and should certainly avoid using it.

There has also been some suggestion that cannabis use can lower IQ and impact on education. An initial study investigated a group of just under 1,000 individuals in Dunedin, New Zealand. Researchers found that individuals who had been heavy users of cannabis during adolescence showed a substantial eight-point drop in IQ between age thirteen, when it was first measured, and age thirty-eight, when it was measured again. This pattern wasn't seen in individuals who first used cannabis after eighteen.

I was involved in some research that used a dataset based in Bristol, UK, to see if the same patterns were seen in these individuals. We found something a little different – in our sample we found that cannabis only predicted lower IQ before we took account of other differences between cannabis users and non-users, in particular behavioural problems and mental health symptoms. We also looked at school results and found the same pattern. So whether cannabis use during adolescence really impacts on IQ is still hotly debated.

There's certainly reason to think that using cannabis during adolescence is more risky than waiting until you're older. Our brains develop a lot during adolescence, and aren't really finished developing until our mid-twenties. The endocannabinoid system is one of the areas that develops during this time – the number of cannabinoid receptors in the brain changes during adolescence.

As such, theoretically it makes sense that cannabis could have more of an impact on IQ, and potentially mental health too, during this time period. But again, it's one of those things that's extremely hard to research, so while we can't definitively say that cannabis is more harmful in adolescence, that doesn't mean it isn't, and delaying when you first try cannabis until after adolescence is over is smart behaviour.

Cannabis can be addictive, and about 9 per cent of users become dependent on it. Cannabis withdrawal can make a person feel anxious and irritable, and can impact on sleep patterns and appetite.

Myths and misconceptions

Cannabis is a gateway drug

Although cannabis use is likely to precede the use of other illicit drugs for most people, this doesn't mean that cannabis causes their use. This is a challenging area to research, and it's possible that the association between cannabis use and later drug use is related to the illicit nature of cannabis.

If you have to buy your cannabis from a dealer on the street, you're exposing yourself to the illicit drug trade, where these other drugs are sold, meaning in all likelihood they'll be more easily accessible than if you'd never used cannabis. The person you buy your cannabis from might themselves sell other drugs, or know someone who does.

? PARTLY TRUE

Queen Victoria used cannabis

Although now seen as predominantly a recreational drug,* cannabis has an unexpected history in the UK as a medicine. It was prescribed in tincture form (extract of cannabis dissolved in alcohol) during Victorian times, as a treatment for what could euphemistically be referred to as women's issues such as period pains and pain during childbirth. There is a persistent story, popular among those advocating for cannabis's decriminalisation, that Queen Victoria herself may have been a user of cannabis, some claiming for period pains or for PMS, others claiming for pain during childbirth.

This myth seems to have come about because one of the doctors in the royal household, Sir John Russell Reynolds, was an advocate for cannabis, prescribing it to individuals for migraine, epilepsy, depression and asthma, among other things. But he wasn't Victoria's personal physician, so the likelihood of him prescribing cannabis to her is slim to none. Not only that, but he didn't begin to work for the household until Victoria herself was sixty years old. So while some Victorians might have been prescribed cannabis, there's no evidence that Victoria herself was.

? PROBABLY MYTH

Cannabis can cure cancer

There are some cannabis advocates who strongly believe that this is the case, and that there is some huge conspiracy among pharmaceutical companies to withhold evidence that cannabis could be revolutionary for cancer prevention and cure. But there simply isn't the evidence to back this up. That said, research into the use of natural and synthetic cannabinoids is currently going on

---

* Although this perception is changing, as medicinal cannabis is becoming better studied and more widely used.

across the globe to look into this more scientifically, and just because we don't have evidence yet doesn't mean cannabis or cannabinoids won't have any use in the treatment of cancer, but we are not at that stage at the moment.

It would be extremely dangerous to stop taking prescribed cancer treatment and move to cannabis – your doctor will be using evidence-based treatments that have been through high levels of scrutiny and testing. This just hasn't happened for cannabis.

There are some ways that cannabis is being used successfully by cancer patients (with an evidence base to back it up). A synthetic cannabinoid mimicking THC was used in the 1980s as a method of reducing chemotherapy-induced nausea. There are now better and safer medications not based on cannabinoids that serve this purpose, so it's not used as much these days, but it does get prescribed occasionally if other medications aren't working for an individual.

In the Netherlands, and some states in the USA, it's possible to get medical cannabis prescribed for the relief of cancer pain in cancer patients with a terminal diagnosis. Here in the UK there are trials ongoing for the use of the Sativex cannabis spray (see below) for such purposes.

? CURRENTLY UNCLEAR

Does cannabis have any medical benefits?

Although cannabis is associated with some harms, cannabis can have some medical benefits. As we've seen, in Victorian times, tincture of cannabis was prescribed for period pains and pain during childbirth, among other things, and only fell out of favour when the syringe was invented. But the medical benefits of cannabis are now being re-harnessed, and more comprehensively interrogated.

Since 2010, Sativex spray has been made available on prescription in the UK and twenty-six other countries, as a treatment for spasticity (a collective term for symptoms such as paralysis, muscle spasms and inability to control limbs properly) in multiple sclerosis. It has to be prescribed by a specialist, and only if other treatments have proved ineffective, but it is available.

What don't we know?

So far I've referred to 'cannabis' as if it's one substance, but this may be misleading. There are lots of different active substances in cannabis. THC is probably the best known and best understood. It's this compound, as detailed above, that has been shown to induce temporary psychotic experiences when intoxicated, for example. But there are other cannabinoids, which could have vastly different effects. One of these – cannabidiol (CBD) – might even be protective against the risk of psychosis.

Initial studies looking at CBD used a similar protocol to the THC intoxication RCTs I described earlier. The difference this time was that half the group were given CBD before they experienced THC, and half were given a placebo. The group given CBD reported substantially lower psychotic-like experiences and memory impairment during their THC intoxication.

More recently, researchers have taken this one step further. In a small-scale proof of concept study, eighty-eight patients with schizophrenia were recruited to take part in a six-week study. Half were given 1,000mg of CBD alongside their usual antipsychotic medication, half a placebo. Crucially both the participants and the researchers didn't know whether they had received CBD – this was a double-blind experiment.

The researchers investigated a number of outcomes, including how the patients themselves felt afterwards, and their symptoms as assessed by their clinicians. At the end of the study, the results suggested that patients given CBD alongside their usual treatment showed a reduction in their psychotic-like experiences, as rated by themselves, and also by their clinicians. This small-scale study can't tell us anything definitive, but it's an intriguing finding that is currently being investigated on a larger scale.

CBD oil is currently being touted as the new miracle cure for everything from chronic pain and stroke recovery to cancer and arthritis. It's also being marketed more generally for its 'wellness' (whatever that means) properties. But don't rush out to your local health food store just yet. At present, the doses you get in commercially available CBD oil are orders of magnitude lower than those given to patients in clinical trials, untested, and unregulated.

I recently interviewed cannabinoid psychopharmacology researcher Dr Amir Englund, and he worries that the CBD being marketed as a wellness product in this way could have negative consequences for research into its potential benefits medicinally. 'People might go out to try these products because they've heard that scientific studies show beneficial effects for different conditions. Then they try these homeopathic-level CBD products and find no benefit, so when a doctor might actually offer them some medical-grade CBD, they'll turn them down.'

It looks like – at present – the effects seen by over-the-counter CBD oil are more akin to the placebo effect than anything inherent in CBD, but ongoing trials are looking at CBD and a number of outcomes, which could be promising in the future.

Having said that, there is growing evidence that medical-grade CBD might be beneficial for certain conditions. So far, the evidence is strongest for certain types of epilepsy, particularly in children, and also in epilepsy that doesn't respond well to other treatments. But much like with other medications, it doesn't seem to work for everyone. Research into CBD in children with epilepsy found that around 12.5 per cent of those given CBD (on top of their current treatment) experienced a halving in the number of seizures they experience, while less than 1 per cent found their seizures stopped completely.

CBD can also interfere with other medications that are prescribed for epilepsy, including clobozam – a benzodiazepine that can be prescribed to control seizures, and sodium valproate. CBD can interfere with liver function, and it can also increase the sedative effects of clobazam. It's not as benign as some may believe.

Ratios of THC and CBD in cannabis cultivated and sold have changed over the past few decades, and it looks like THC levels have risen as CBD levels have fallen. While not universally true, in most instances 'skunk' cannabis seems to have a particularly imbalanced ratio of these compounds, with many strains of skunk containing only trace amounts of CBD and high levels of THC. If it is the case that THC might induce psychosis but CBD is protective, it's easy to see why these changes in relative levels could be problematic.

Some have suggested that these changes in cannabis's make-up might mean that the earlier studies looking at cannabis and mental health in previous decades are no longer applicable, and might underestimate harm. Others think this is a problem regulation could solve – if you knew and could 'choose' the strength of cannabis that you use, and the relative levels of these cannabinoids, maybe this could help minimise the risk of harm.

Unfortunately, evidence gathered from places where cannabis has been legalised suggests this might not be the case. The changing legal status of cannabis across the world has allowed researchers to be able to look at whether the type of cannabis people use is different under prohibition versus regulation.

A study conducted in Washington state, where the first licensed retailer opened in July 2014, investigated over 30 million cannabis sales in the state, between July 2014 and September 2016. They found that extremely high-THC cannabis products remain the most popular (often with higher THC levels than those seen in samples taken from the street in the UK), disputing the idea that it is only prohibition that pushes up THC concentrations, and given choice people would prefer lower-THC products.

Cannabis products themselves are changing, too. In recent years, cannabis concentrates and 'dabbing' have become more popular. These are created by extracting THC (and potentially other cannabinoids) by using a solvent such as butane. The resulting product is a sticky oil, sometimes called wax, shatter or butane hash oil (BHO), and generally known as 'a dab'.

Dabbing is the process of heating up and inhaling these concentrates, which are often exceptionally high potency – the same Washington study also looked at concentrates, and found that while THC levels in cannabis plants purchased was around 20 per cent, in cannabis concentrates the levels were much higher, peaking at around 70 per cent, but reaching over 90 per cent in some samples.

In Washington state they currently make up 21 per cent of cannabis sales in the state, increasing their market share by over 140 per cent between October 2014 and September 2016. Whether this pattern is the same in places where cannabis remains illicit is harder to ascertain. What the impact of the growing popularity of these products will be is yet to be known, in terms of health, and mental health risks.

CHAPTER 6

Cigarettes

NICOTINE

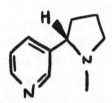

What is it? Nicotine is found in tobacco plants – cigarettes are
dried tobacco leaves and additives wrapped in paper,
usually with a filter made of cellulose acetate.

Type of drug: Nicotine is a stimulant.

Popularity: Falling out of favour now, but still legal pretty much
everywhere.

How consumed: Cigarettes are smoked, nicotine can also be
consumed in patches, sprays and inhalators.

Timescale: Nicotine reaches the brain within seconds, and the
effect lasts for a few minutes.

Some effects: Increased heart rate, blood pressure. Reduction
in withdrawal symptoms for dependent smokers.

WELL – TOBACCO really, I'm cheating by calling this chapter
'Cigarettes', but alphabetically it just works!

Tobacco, the dried leaf that is smoked in cigarettes, cigars and
pipes, and taken in various other forms such as snus and chewing

tobacco, has been used as a recreational drug for hundreds, if not thousands of years. The World Health Organisation states that the tobacco plant was first cultivated in the Americas in around 6000 BC. There is evidence that indigenous Americans were smoking tobacco as far back as 1 BC, as well as using tobacco enemas. There's some suggestion that tobacco was used ceremonially at this time.

Christopher Columbus brought tobacco from the Americas to Europe, and its popularity spread quickly across the globe from that point. In the eighteenth century, snuff was a popular method for consumption of tobacco, while in the nineteenth century, the cigar overtook it. Cigarettes as a method for smoking became popular during World War One, when they were included as part of British soldiers' ration packs – once cigarettes could be manufactured mechanically and at a large scale, their popularity rose dramatically.

Two in three regular smokers will have started smoking before the age of eighteen, and smoking is illegal in this age group in the UK and many other countries around the world. The percentage of current smokers who want to quit is similarly high (around two in three current smokers report wanting to stop smoking). People who smoke report that it relieves stress, and can make them feel calmer and more relaxed. But is this really the case?

What is it?

Nicotine is the active compound in tobacco. Its molecular structure is similar to the neurotransmitter acetylcholine, and it binds to acetylcholine receptors in the brain, mimicking the action of the neurotransmitter and giving nicotine its mild stimulant properties (more later). It also has an influence on dopamine (a neurotransmitter that is thought to be involved in reward and pleasure). Because nicotine is the active compound in tobacco, people often mistakenly believe that it's nicotine that is responsible for the harms caused by smoking cigarettes.

Nicotine can be habit-forming, but interestingly there's something unique about cigarettes that makes the nicotine in them particularly addictive. Because of the chemical balance (pH) of tobacco in cigarettes, the smoke has to be breathed into the lungs in order for the nicotine to be absorbed into the blood. This is in contrast with other tobacco products like chewing tobacco or even cigars, where the nicotine is absorbed mostly through the lining of the mouth. When nicotine is absorbed through the lungs, it gets into the bloodstream, and then the brain, within seconds, while absorption through the mouth is a much slower route. The quicker a substance reaches the brain, the higher the risk of dependence on it.

What are the short-term effects?

While there's no real intoxication effect of cigarettes, if a person is not used to nicotine a cigarette can make them feel sick or dizzy. Nicotine reaches the brain within seconds, and the effect of nicotine wears off within a few minutes. Smoking a cigarette raises your heart rate. If a person is a regular smoker and dependent on nicotine, then smoking a cigarette can bring a person out of withdrawal. Nicotine withdrawal is characterised by feelings of anxiety, irritability, headaches and difficulty concentrating.

Many researchers think the reason that smokers report feeling lower anxiety and stress levels after smoking a cigarette is because of the alleviation of these withdrawal effects – this seems likely, as long-term use of cigarettes is associated with higher levels of depression and anxiety.

What are the longer-term effects?

The physical health impacts of cigarettes have been known for well over half a century. Cigarettes are responsible for the premature deaths of two in three regular users, according to recent figures from the UK and the USA. Smoking causes lung cancer, and at least thirteen other types of cancer, to varying degrees. Cancer Research UK estimates that smoking causes a quarter of all cancer deaths in the UK, and nearly one in five cancer cases. Aside from cancers, smoking also increases the risk of a variety of other heart and lung diseases.

There has been some suggestion that smoking, or nicotine in particular, might be beneficial for Parkinson's disease. The charity Parkinson's UK has even funded research looking into this. However, as yet the evidence is thin on the ground, and there's some reason to believe that this seemingly positive association might be misleading. Given that so many smokers are killed by their habit, the smokers who survive long enough to be at risk of Parkinson's disease might be an unusually hardy bunch, so it could be this aspect of their genetic or environmental make-up, rather than the nicotine they are consuming, that's protective against Parkinson's.

Elderly smokers represent a really interesting population to research for this reason – if we can identify why these individuals don't succumb to smoking-related illnesses, this might be hugely beneficial for designing treatments for others.

Myths and misconceptions

Nicotine is extremely harmful

While nicotine is the addictive substance in cigarettes, it's not the really harmful part of them. The process of burning tobacco releases carbon monoxide, hydrogen cyanide, at least seventy known carcinogens, and a variety of other chemicals. Nicotine is addictive, but specifically in cigarettes rather than in other forms, as discussed above. Nicotine is a mild stimulant and has an effect on health probably more akin to coffee than speed – it increases your heart rate and blood pressure slightly.

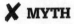 **MYTH**

Menthol cigarettes are safer / Menthol cigarettes are more harmful

There is disagreement even among the myths surrounding menthol cigarettes – tobacco cigarettes flavoured with mint. There has been less research conducted on menthol cigarettes compared to regular cigarettes, but there's no evidence to suggest they are any more or less harmful – it seems likely that they're just as harmful as regular tobacco.

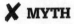 **MYTH**

Roll-ups or 'natural tobacco' are less harmful than other cigarettes

It's a common belief that rolling tobacco contains fewer of the harmful chemicals and components found in machine-made cigarettes. When questioned about it, between 21 per cent and 40 per cent of roll-up smokers in Canada, Australia, the UK and the USA said they smoke roll-ups because they thought they were healthier than manufactured cigarettes.

This is a myth. Some studies have found that rolling tobacco actually contains more additives by weight than factory-made cigarettes, and one animal study suggested that rolling tobacco was more addictive, although this was only a small study, meaning the results might not be very reliable. But there are perhaps some reasons to believe this increased addictiveness could be the case in humans, too.

Although repeated nicotine use can lead to dependence on cigarettes, a lot of the addiction can be psychological. Smokers have their 'ritual' of smoking – be this going outside, the act of buying cigarettes, or even removing them from the packet and lighting them. For people who smoke roll-ups, this ritual can be extended. The act of building the cigarette, the anticipation of being about to smoke it, maybe this increases the reward experience of smoking, and therefore the addictive properties. Of course, this wasn't what was happening in the animal study (unless these were some particularly dextrous mice who were rolling their own).

✗ MYTH

Light or low-tar cigarettes are less harmful than other cigarettes

You may have noticed that there's no such thing as Marlboro Lights anymore. Tobacco companies are no longer allowed to market cigarettes as 'light' or 'low tar', since light cigarettes were found to be no less harmful than regular cigarettes. And this was due to the difference between humans and machines.

Light cigarettes, first introduced in the 1970s, never actually contained less tar than other cigarettes. The alterations were made to the filter: more ventilation holes were put in it to allow more smoke to escape before it was inhaled into the lungs. The cigarette paper itself was also made out of more porous material for the same reason, the idea being that fewer harmful particles would be breathed in.

These newly designed cigarettes were tested by organisations such as the Federal Trade Commission in the USA, using machines that 'smoked' the cigarettes and took readings of the tar yield, and lo and behold, this new design yielded lower tar levels. The machines 'inhaled' lower levels of harmful smoke. But humans aren't machines, and they altered their smoking patterns, moving their mouths further over the filter, squeezing at the filters and dragging more deeply on the cigarettes. Experimental research has since borne this out – smokers get just as much tar from light cigarettes as from other brands.

But just because the tobacco industry are not allowed to call their products low tar any more, doesn't mean they don't try and get the (incorrect) message across in other ways. In countries where they are allowed to, many companies still use descriptive words or packaging colour to imply reduced harm (for example, gold or red).

✗ MYTH

Using a hookah pipe or shisha is less harmful than smoking cigarettes

Shishas, hookahs, waterpipes, hubble bubble – these are all names to describe the practice of smoking tobacco through a water chamber, via a long hose-like mouthpiece. Flavoured tobacco is placed under a foil-covered platform at the top of the bowl, then covered with hot charcoal. Users breathe through the hose, drawing smoke through the water and into their mouths. Shisha is sociable, with pipes having multiple hoses, or hoses being passed around.

Waterpipe use is on the rise in the UK, particularly among teenagers and young adults. And there are some worrying misconceptions about its safety. Many people, for example, do not realise that the flavoured tobacco smoked through a shisha pipe is still tobacco. It is possible to get non-tobacco herbal mixtures to smoke, but these are less common than flavoured tobacco. The herbal mixtures still release a number of the same toxins found in tobacco smoke when burnt, and there is benzene and carbon monoxide released by the burning charcoal that is also inhaled.

Some erroneously believe that the water purifies the smoke somehow – there is no evidence to suggest this. In 2016, a systematic review of the literature on shisha pipes was undertaken, and researchers found that use of the pipes was linked to many of the same illnesses and risks as smoking cigarettes – respiratory disease, lung cancer, mouth cancer, poor mental health, low birth-weight of offspring and cardiovascular disease levels were all increased compared to those who did not use shisha, to name a few health outcomes.

Unfortunately, no studies to date have compared risks from shisha use directly to risks from using cigarettes – it might be that using shisha is less harmful than smoking, but even if that were the case, this could be because of the nature of use. Shisha is used socially, and at special occasions, rather than being used daily in the way cigarettes are. However, it might be that there are increased risks from shisha compared to cigarettes – for example, as the smoke is cooled by the water, it is easier to hold it in the lungs for longer, potentially increasing exposure to the harmful compounds found in tobacco smoke.

As yet we just don't know, but the idea that shisha is less harmful than cigarettes is not true – the evidence to date suggests that, puff for puff, shisha is broadly equivalent in risk to tobacco cigarettes.

 MYTH

Cutting down smoking will reduce the levels of harm from smoking

It seems hard to believe that this isn't the case, but cutting down the number of cigarettes you smoke doesn't necessarily reduce the risk of smoking-related harm. This is connected to the myth above – if a person is used to getting a certain amount of nicotine in a day, then if they smoke fewer cigarettes, they're likely to draw more deeply, take more puffs, and hold the smoke in their lungs longer for the cigarettes they do smoke. And also, of course, tobacco is harmful even at lower levels. Psychologically, cutting down is a great first step in the quit process, but in terms of harm reduction, quitting is really the only way.

? PARTLY TRUE

Everyone dies of something, so why not smoking? Smoking just means I'll miss the last few years, which are the worst ones

This is a frequent comment I've heard when giving talks or chatting to libertarians on the internet. And it's true that we will all die of something. However, it's not true to say that smoking means you'll miss the old and ill years at the end of life. Smoking-related illnesses and deaths are often extremely unpleasant, protracted, and earlier than non-tobacco related deaths. Yes, you might miss the later years of your life if you smoke, but you might also find yourself seriously ill at an earlier age, and you might lose your life many years earlier than you would otherwise.

✗ MYTH

I've smoked for years, I've already damaged my health – there's no point quitting

With all the doom and gloom in the above myth, and how notoriously difficult it is to stop smoking, it's not surprising that some smokers will presume that the damage has already been done, so there's no point in giving up. However, a growing body of research has found that the health benefits of stopping smoking apply even to the most hardened smoker. Within months of stopping smoking, a person will have a lower risk of stroke and heart disease than they did while they were a smoker. No matter how long you've smoked, there are benefits from quitting.

 MYTH

What don't we know?

You might think that we know all there is to know about cigarettes and tobacco. We've known for more than half a century that smoking causes lung cancer, and the physical effects of smoking are fairly well understood. But there is still a lot that we don't know. For example, why do some people find it easy to stop smoking, while others really struggle?

There's evidence that smoking behaviour is partly genetic. Slight differences in a person's genotype (their DNA code) predict how heavily they will smoke, if they are a smoker, and these small differences can affect smoking behaviour up to the level of a couple of cigarettes extra per day. This might go some way to explaining why it's easier for some to give up than others, and could even represent a method to work out how to help a person to stop. If your dependence is stronger, maybe it would benefit you to have counselling support, use nicotine-replacement therapy, or even take medication to help (called pharmacotherapy), rather than trying to give up cold turkey.

The other emerging area of research that I'm really interested in is trying to understand why smoking rates are so much higher in populations with mental health difficulties. We understand the physical effects of tobacco so well, but we're much less sure about why these associations come about.

At the beginning of this chapter I mentioned that smoking is associated with depression and anxiety. But why is this? Does smoking somehow increase the risk? Do people who suffer from these conditions take up smoking for some reason? Or does something else that happens earlier in life, or even something more innate, predict both a likelihood to smoke and risk of poor mental health?

It's really hard to tease this out. Smoking is also seen at far higher levels in people with psychotic disorders or schizophrenia. Historically it's been assumed this is because nicotine might alleviate some of the negative side-effects of anti-psychotic medication, which can be quite severe. But smoking often predates a person getting ill, which might call this into question.

Also, really interestingly, when researchers investigated the genetics of schizophrenia risk in a huge study of over 200,000 individuals, one of the 100 or so genetic variants (a single letter change in the DNA code of some individuals compared to others) that predicts risk of schizophrenia has also been found, in a completely different study, to predict the number of cigarettes per day that daily smokers are likely to smoke. The same single letter change of DNA predicts both heaviness of smoking, and risk of schizophrenia.

What might this mean? Well, it could just be a coincidence – we don't really understand how tiny genetic changes like this might lead to differences in risk of behaviours like smoking, or in diseases like schizophrenia. This variant might be doing nothing at all. Intriguingly, though, another possibility might be that this variant doesn't have anything to do with schizophrenia, but is seen in the schizophrenia study because it predicts heaviness of smoking, and smoking is seen at such high levels in individuals with schizophrenia.*

It might even be evidence that smoking might increase the risk of schizophrenia – but we can't tell from these findings alone. I don't think the evidence is convincing yet that smoking increases the risk of schizophrenia, and it's also worth thinking about the size of the risk, too. It's miniscule in comparison to the risk of smoking-related diseases such as lung cancer. But that doesn't mean the link between smoking and mental health isn't important.

As I've mentioned, smoking is seen at far higher levels in people with schizophrenia than national averages (recent estimates suggest around 60 per cent of patients with schizophrenia are smokers), and people with the disorder have a lower life-expectancy than average as well, often from diseases that are linked to smoking.

Finally, as we have seen prevalence of smoking reduce in countries like the UK, we've begun to notice that this might be increasing health inequality.

Estimates suggest that in 2018, 14.9 per cent of the adult population in the UK were smokers. In the 1950s, it was estimated that almost half the adult population of the UK smoked. This then dropped gradually over the following decades, with decreases speeding up more recently as policies were put in place to improve education and limit advertising of tobacco products. But smoking

---

* In fact, this variant is also seen in genetic studies of the predictors of lung cancer. And we know this is due to its link to smoking, because when the genetics of lung cancer were investigated in non-smokers only, this variant was no longer associated with the disease. I really wanted to investigate this with schizophrenia, but unfortunately there are currently no large enough datasets available where schizophrenia, genetics, and smoking status have been measured.

is becoming more and more socially patterned, as people with better support networks are finding it easier to stop smoking than those without the support.

This seems counterintuitive at first – you'd think that reducing the number of people smoking (we've seen huge drops in smoking prevalence in the UK over the last few decades) would improve health. But overarching numbers can be misleading and hide the patterns in sub-groups of people – and this really suggests that more support is needed for people from lower socio-economic backgrounds, before health inequality gets any wider.

CHAPTER 7

Cocaine

What is it? Found in the coca leaf in western South America.
Type of drug: Stimulant.
Popularity: A popular illicit drug in the UK, the second most
used after cannabis. Currently dangerously pure, and deaths
from cocaine are on the rise.
How consumed: Leaves can be chewed, powder can be
swallowed, or snorted, crack can be smoked or injected.
Timescale: Varies by method of consumption; the quicker it
reaches the brain, the quicker it wears off.
Some effects: Increases confidence, heart rate, body
temperature, can cause insomnia, heart palpitations.

COCAINE HAS SOMETHING of a reputation. If you ask people to
name 'a hard drug', cocaine might be the first they think of. And
intoxication on cocaine is often used as short-hand for any loud
irritating group of people you might encounter – 'Oh, I saw a
load of coked-up businessmen in the bar.' Whether every loud

confident group of posh men are really on cocaine is up for debate, but that's the reputation the drug has.

Cocaine is certainly one of the more popular illicit drugs in the UK. The European Monitoring Centre for Drugs and Drug Addiction estimate that 2.7 per cent of UK sixteen- to fifty-nine-year-olds took cocaine (with 2.6 per cent of those taking powdered cocaine) between 2017 and 2018. Cocaine is also an illicit drug that constantly makes headlines in the UK press. At the end of 2018, the then Home Secretary Sajid Javid pledged to crack down (no pun intended) on middle-class cocaine users, blaming them for the rise in knife crime being seen in London and elsewhere in the UK.*

Earlier in 2018, the media was awash (again, I'm sorry) with stories about cocaine getting into London's rivers and streams, and impacting on endangered eel populations that live there – causing them to become hyperactive, to suffer muscle wasting, and impacting their gills and their hormone levels. And while I was writing this chapter, Noel Gallagher made headlines by declaring that cocaine is 'boring'.

Thanks for your input, Noel, but sadly the press disagreed and wrote a frankly unnecessary number of articles about his statement. But alongside these puff pieces, deaths from cocaine in England and Wales are at the highest level since data began being collected, in 1993.

---

* I was invited on the BBC's *Victoria Derbyshire* programme to talk about this at the time. I pointed out that evidence collated by the Advisory Council for the Misuse of Drugs has shown that punitive punishments for drug use are not very effectual in getting people to stop, even if the middle class was a sensible target for intervention (which it might not be – the people who need the most help are the people experiencing the most harms from drugs, which probably isn't that group).

What is it?

Cocaine – or benzoylmethylecgonine to give it its chemical name – is a drug that can be taken in many forms, via a number of different methods. And this can mean that the same underlying substance can have a variety of effects. Broadly, cocaine is a stimulant, an upper, so it'll do all the things that stimulants will do. But a person chewing coca leaf will have a markedly different intoxication experience, and risk of dependence, compared to someone inhaling crack cocaine vapour. Similarly, the appeal of snorting powder cocaine might not be the same as the appeal of crack, or of coca leaf.

What are the different types of cocaine?

Cocaine itself is found naturally in coca leaves, which grow in western South American countries such as Bolivia, Argentina and Peru. The leaves of the plant are mixed with lime (by which I mean calcium hydroxide or calcium carbonate, rather than 'coca leaves with a twist of lime'), or another alkaloid substance that allows it to be absorbed through the lining of the mouth. The leaves are chewed into a wad, which a person will tuck in-between their gum and cheek and leave there, sucking the juices out of it.

Coca leaves can also be steeped in hot water to make coca tea, a drink particularly popular in the Andes mountain range – indeed climbers have reported being encouraged to drink it to reduce altitude sickness (although whether it is effective in this regard has never been properly investigated).

Cocaine can also be extracted from coca leaves, and it is in these forms that cocaine is more commonly used around the rest of the world. If someone refers to cocaine, they'll usually be talking about cocaine hydrochloride, or powder cocaine. Cocaine prepared in this way is usually snorted (nasal insufflation is the scientific term for this, fact fans). Often this will happen through a rolled-up bank note, or another small tube (some people use biros with the ink part removed, or unused tampon applicators). The cocaine powder will coat the inside of the nasal passage and be absorbed through the mucous membranes into the bloodstream. What isn't absorbed will then be picked up in mucus and 'drip' down the back of a person's throat to be swallowed.

Cocaine can also be prepared for smoking (actually heating and inhaling the vapour, rather than burning and smoking) and injecting. A final preparation of cocaine is called freebase. This is cocaine sulphate – cocaine without the hydrochloride found in powder cocaine. It's consumed in the same way as crack cocaine, and often the terms are used interchangeably.

Crack cocaine is broadly similar to freebase, although usually contains adulterants, so is less pure than freebase. It's often prepared using baking soda and water. It looks like an oily or plastic-y waxy rock (why it's often called a rock of crack). Crack is usually smoked through a small glass pipe. It can also be injected if dissolved in an acid.

The method by which cocaine is consumed will impact on how quickly it gets into the brain, and therefore how soon after consumption a person will start to feel intoxicated. As you might expect, injecting a drug means it reaches the brain very quickly – within seconds. The length of intoxication is correspondingly short, with the acute effects of cocaine wearing off within about fifteen to twenty minutes. Inhaling a vapour is almost as fast – the vapour is inhaled into the lungs and so is transferred into the bloodstream within a few seconds.

If a person snorts cocaine, it takes slightly longer to get into the bloodstream – an individual will start to feel the effect approximately five minutes after snorting. When cocaine is snorted, it also constricts the blood vessels in the nose, meaning absorption is slightly slowed. Intoxication via this method tends to last around half an hour.

Chewing coca leaves is the slowest method by which to consume cocaine, taking about half an hour to enter the bloodstream, and the intoxication experience, while milder, will last substantially longer.

What are the short-term effects?

Intoxication on cocaine can make an individual feel confident and upbeat – it's a stimulant, so it can increase alertness, as well as causing feelings of euphoria, a clear head and a good mood. Like other stimulants, cocaine increases an individual's heart rate, and raises their body temperature. It's also an appetite suppressant, like other stimulants.

As a person increases their dose of cocaine, it can cause them to become sweaty, to get a dry mouth, and there's some suggestion it can make individuals more aggressive (this could be linked to increased feelings of confidence, or feelings of invincibility – a lack of the social inhibitions a person might feel when sober). As the dose increases yet further, people can experience headaches, insomnia and nausea. Individuals who snort cocaine can experience nasal irritation. Individuals who inject cocaine sometimes report a sudden tinnitus accompanying the initial intoxication experience.

Taking too much cocaine can be extremely dangerous. A person might experience palpitations, or even seizures. Hyperthermia, where body temperature increases, is also a possibility, as well as a heightened risk of a heart attack. Psychologically, paranoia, hallucinations and panic attacks are possible.

What are the longer-term effects?

Long-term use of cocaine confers a number of risks on an individual. If a person is snorting cocaine, they run the risk of lasting damage to their nasal passage and septum, including painful nasal ulcers, and the potential of a perforated septum (discussed in more detail below). People inhaling cocaine vapour are at risk of respiratory problems including asthma and emphysema. Not only that, but the melting point of crack is extremely high, and crack pipes are often short because the vapour only remains potent for a short amount of time. This means the pipes and vapour are extremely hot when they meet a person's mouth, so there is a risk of blistering on the lips from regular inhalation of crack.

There is evidence that cocaine is addictive, but as you might expect, how likely a person is to experience dependence will be influenced by a number of factors, including the method of consumption. A usual rule of thumb is that the quicker a substance takes effect, and the shorter the intoxication experience, the higher the risk of developing dependence. Smoking or injecting cocaine regularly is therefore more risky in terms of dependence than snorting, which is itself more risky than chewing coca leaves. People who stop taking cocaine after using it regularly report experiencing withdrawal symptoms, including low mood and irritability.

Long-term use of cocaine has been linked to a number of mental health problems, including depression, anxiety and paranoia. Much like the links between mental health and other substances, these associations are seen in observational studies, so it's difficult to say with any certainty whether the cocaine use causes the mental health problems, or whether people with mental health problems are more likely to use cocaine. It's also perfectly possible that both of those statements could be true.

Animal studies have found some evidence that chronic cocaine use might cause brain damage, particularly to the white matter of the brain. In humans, this has been harder to research. There's some suggestion that this brain damage might occur because cocaine narrows blood vessels, so might reduce blood flow in the brain. This narrowing of blood vessels might also increase a regular user's risk of heart attacks and stroke, although again the evidence for this is mostly based on anecdote and case reports rather than large-scale studies. It's also possible that liver damage might result if an individual takes cocaine very regularly, without allowing their body to recover between uses.

As with many substances, cocaine is a drug that is rarely taken on its own. But mixing cocaine with other substances can lead to unexpected risks, above and beyond those of each substance individually. Taking cocaine with other stimulants can put extra pressure on the heart and increase the possibility of heart attacks. Taking cocaine with depressants can result in 'masking', where the stimulant effects of cocaine might hide the depressant effects of something like alcohol or heroin. This can make overdosing more likely, as a person isn't able to assess how the drugs are affecting them properly. And with alcohol there is an additional risk.

When cocaine and alcohol mix, a by-product called cocaethylene is created. Some researchers have suggested that cocaethylene is responsible for increased heart attacks and liver problems in individuals who have co-used alcohol and cocaine for a number of years. Other researchers are not so sure – because taking cocaine and alcohol can mask the effects of the other, it might be the case that people who use both, on average and over the course of their drug-taking lives, consume higher levels of both cocaine and alcohol, and so these increased harms might be due to higher doses, rather than this new chemical. Either way, taking both together increases the risk above and beyond taking either substance by itself.

Another popular combination with high risks is known as a

speedball – mixing cocaine and heroin, and either snorting or injecting the combination. As we've discussed above, mixing a stimulant and a depressant can mask the effect of both, meaning a person can feel more alert and awake than they usually would after taking heroin, because of the stimulant effect of cocaine. This makes the risk of overdose more likely.

Speedballs have been implicated by the media in a number of high-profile deaths, including River Phoenix, John Belushi and Philip Seymour Hoffman. That said, the media can often present a somewhat warped picture of risk of harm from substances – individual cases can mislead, as there may be other underlying risks not known about that could also be at play.

We know very little about the number of individuals who mix cocaine and heroin in this way, and so it's hard to estimate the level of risk very accurately. From our understanding of how stimulants and depressants interact, we can certainly be sure that mixing them will increase risk of overdose, and overdosing on cocaine or heroin can have severe, potentially fatal consequences.

Cocaine can be particularly dangerous to use for pregnant women. Cocaine use during pregnancy has been linked to problems with the foetus, such as low birth weight, smaller head circumference and generally being smaller. It's also linked to risk of miscarriage and of sudden infant death syndrome. However, given it's rare for people to use only one drug, it's difficult to be really sure how many of these effects are specific to cocaine.

In the 1980s there was a large panic about 'crack babies' (an awful term) – with the suggestion that women dependent on crack cocaine were giving birth to babies that would have reduced intelligence and social skills. This moral panic seems to have been hugely exaggerated, but there do seem to be some mild impairments in children exposed to cocaine *in utero*, such as behaviour problems and small deficits in some aspects of information processing and attention.

The possibility of confounding is high here, though – children regularly exposed to cocaine during pregnancy are likely to have different upbringings to those who were not in lots of ways, and this might also impact on their behaviour and attention.

Myths and misconceptions

There are a whole load of myths and misconceptions that exist around cocaine – probably because it's one of the most commonly used illicit drugs, usually ranking second in popularity after cannabis. Here are some of the more common ones.

The addictive properties of cocaine depend on method of use

This is fairly accurate, as we've discussed above. You're at a higher risk of developing dependence from cocaine use if you inject or smoke it, although snorting it also means the drug will get into your bloodstream quite quickly, meaning risk of dependence is still rather high for that method of consumption.

 TRUE

If you use cocaine once you can/will become addicted

This is said of a lot of substances, but even the highest estimates suggest that of people who use cocaine, about 50 per cent will develop addiction – and most estimates are substantially lower than that, meaning it's likely that at least half of all people who try cocaine will not develop dependence. You can't become dependent on a substance if you have never tried it – and everyone who develops dependence will have used a substance at least once, that's fairly obvious. And the first time experiencing a substance can be a significant step on a pathway towards addiction – but it is by no means guaranteed.

Addiction is defined as repeating and persisting in a behaviour, in the face of potential or actual harm caused by it, and changing your life around it. Clearly this cannot happen after just one use.

 MYTH

Cocaine will rot your septum

The septum is the piece of skin between the two nostril holes in your nose. In 2000 in the UK, the tabloid press posted shocking pictures of an actress in the popular soap opera *EastEnders*, which seemed to show her septum was missing. Cue headlines about cocaine rotting your nose. Cocaine will not rot your septum, but it can lead to it disintegrating if you are a really heavy cocaine user. If you snort coke regularly, the advice is to wash your nasal passages frequently, though it is also highly advisable to take regular breaks from using cocaine to allow your nasal passages to recover too!

 MYTH

Cocaine sobers you up

While the effects of cocaine on top of alcohol might make a person feel like they're sobering up, this is not the case. Taking cocaine after you've had alcohol might make you feel like you're more sober, but the effects of the cocaine are merely masking the alcohol intoxication. And as cocaine intoxication lasts for only a short time, once the cocaine wears off, you'll feel just as drunk, or even more so if you've carried on drinking.

 MYTH

Cocaine is vegan

Although cocaine is made from a plant, that doesn't mean no animals are harmed in its production. Because of its illicit nature there are no regulations on crop production, and this can mean deforestation and pollution from the dumping of by-products of cocaine production.

There's some evidence (although it's hard to quantify this) that herbicides are used to a higher degree when growing cocaine than when growing other crops in the region where it is grown – so even if you still want to argue it's vegan, it is certainly not organic! And it's also not an ethical product, given the huge human and environmental impact associated with cocaine production and distribution.

? UNCLEAR

If your white powder numbs your mouth when you dab it on your gums, it's definitely cocaine

MDMA white powder will make your gum feel numb, ketamine powder will make your gum feel numb – this isn't a good way to distinguish between substances. And a 'white powder' could contain any number of other adulterants. Getting your drugs tested to find out what's in them before taking the drug is the only way to better understand them.

This is easier said than done – at the moment in the UK, at some music festivals there is an organisation called The Loop to whom you can take your drugs to be tested. In Wales there is a postal drug testing service called WEDINOS. It's also possible to buy kits online that can test for the presence or absence of specific substances. However, these can give a false sense of security, because they can't tell you everything that's in the powder.

These kits only test for the presence or absence of specific substances – anything else in there will go undetected.

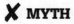 **MYTH**

You can't overdose on cocaine
Er, yes – you absolutely can. It's really dangerous to take too much cocaine, and it can be fatal.

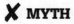 **MYTH**

Does cocaine have any medical uses?

Cocaine has a fascinating history. Although used for thousands of years by communities in the Andes mountains and the Amazon rainforest in the form of coca leaves, cocaine was first extracted from the leaves by scientists in Europe in the mid-1800s. One scientist in Germany noticed that the powder made his tongue feel numb when he tasted it (this seems to be somewhat of a theme – European scientists experimenting on themselves with substances they've extracted from plants; I don't think that happens so much these days . . .).

An ophthalmologist in Austria experimented with the use of cocaine as a local anaesthetic for cataract surgery. The more popular anaesthetics of the time, such as ether or chloroform, had a tendency to make people throw up, so they were not ideal for delicate eye surgery! But cocaine as an anaesthetic did not last long, as patients began dying of accidental overdose in the operating theatre.

Sigmund Freud, later famous for an obsession with penises and wanting to have sex with his mother,* was very interested in understanding the nature of cocaine, before he turned to psychoanalysis. Indeed, his first major publication was entitled *Uber Coca*. In it, he argued that cocaine could be used to treat morphine and alcohol addiction. As you can probably imagine from the contents of this chapter, Freud was not wholly correct in this assumption.

Not only did he end up apparently becoming dependent on cocaine for a number of years, he also recommended it to his friend Ernst Fleischl-Marxow, who was at the time dependent on morphine. It seems that the cocaine did not help Ernst to reduce or stop his morphine use, and he ended up using both, with some reports suggesting he was injecting both (the extremely dangerous 'speedball' mentioned earlier). Whether Ernst was able to stop using morphine or cocaine is unclear, but he passed away around seven years after Freud first introduced him to cocaine, aged forty-five.

Around the same time as cocaine was being investigated for its medical benefits, it was also being marketed as a wellness product. 'Vin Mariani' was red wine and cocaine (again, a combination not recommended, as discussed above) developed by a French chemist called Angelo Mariani in 1863. The adverts for it claimed it 'fortifies and refreshes body and brain' and 'restores health and vitality', and it became popular across Europe where it was sold.

Across the Atlantic in the USA, a pharmacist called John Stith Pemberton founded Coca-Cola in 1886. The beverage was initially made from cocaine and sugary syrup, and sold at soda fountains accessible only to white Americans. When the drink became available in bottles, in 1899, it was available to anyone regardless of their race or class. The company removed cocaine

---

* Or something . . .

from their drinks in 1903, and some claim this was racially motivated – many newspapers and politicians reported or believed that black people who had taken cocaine were particularly dangerous.

This racist view was further evidenced in the 1980s, when crack cocaine use became more common. Punishments for possession of crack were 100 times greater than they were for powder cocaine, which impacted on African Americans as they were more likely to use crack. In 2010, the Fair Sentencing Act reduced this discrepancy, but punishments for crack cocaine possession remained eighteen times higher than for powder cocaine.

CHAPTER 8
DMT/Ayahuasca

DMT

What is it? DMT is found naturally in plants, or synthesised powder, can also be found in a drink – ayahuasca.

Type of drug: Psychedelic.

Popularity: Amazonian ayahuasca rituals are growing in popularity, although still quite niche.

How consumed: DMT powder can be snorted, smoked or injected. Ayahuasca is drunk.

Timescale: Short-lasting compared to other psychedelics if snorted, can last around an hour; if drunk can last 4 to 10 hours.

Some effects: Perceptual alterations, time distortion, vivid colours and shapes, some people vomit.

WOULD YOU LIKE to come face to face with your 'shadow self'? Do you want to 'gain access to deeper layers of your consciousness' and 'reflect intensively on yourself and on your life'? This is how ayahuasca 'ritual' packages are marketed on the internet.

The substance has become extremely popular in recent years, with young people wanting to find themselves travelling to countries like the Netherlands, with their tolerant drug policies, or places like Peru, Colombia, Ecuador or Brazil, where these rituals originated, to experience a potentially life-changing trip.

If a person decides to go on one of these retreats, this is the type of thing they might experience. Ritual is important from the offset – participants might be asked to remove footwear, or dress in a certain way before entering the space where the intoxication will take place. The communal aspect might be highlighted, with people perhaps being asked to share their story or their expectations within the group, or to take part in communal singing or chanting.

There will usually be a guide or leader in charge of the ceremony. They might recite incantations, play instruments, or use incense to enhance the atmosphere. Many websites offering ayahuasca retreats will boast that their shamans are native Peruvians. Ceremonies can last for many hours, and often involve vomiting, or purging, as part of them.

It used to be that ayahuasca consumption was reserved for the shaman – they would use the substance and the resultant intoxication experiences to treat individual ailments or concerns, or to provide wisdom about issues impacting on the group or society more broadly. Nowadays, ayahuasca rituals are open to anyone who will pay.

What is it?

DMT (N, N-dimethyltryptamine) is a psychedelic, and like psilocybin, it occurs in nature. It is found in a number of plants in South and Latin America, where it's been used for many years, as snuff inhaled up the nose, or as ayahuasca – a drink where a DMT-containing plant is mixed with another plant and brewed (more on this below). At a molecular level, its structure is very similar to the neurotransmitter serotonin.

Some people refer to DMT as a 'businessman's trip' – it's a much shorter-lasting intoxication experience than LSD, where intoxication can sometimes last a whole day. It's unclear for how many years DMT has been used in the Americas, but European explorers witnessed the use of snuffs and brews by indigenous populations in the 1800s. The chemical compound DMT was also synthesised in the 1930s, quite separately, and it wasn't until many years later that it was realised that these were the same compounds, or that the synthesised DMT was a powerful psychedelic drug.

For some, the appeal of DMT is that it is 'more natural' than LSD, being extracted from a plant, but more powerful or intense than magic mushrooms (psilocybin). It's perhaps appealing because of its historical (and current) use in rituals.

If DMT is swallowed, enzymes in our stomachs called mono-amine oxidases will neutralise the molecule before it can cause any intoxicating effect. However, if DMT is mixed with mono-amine oxidase inhibitors, these enzymes can be prevented from having an impact, and it will be possible to experience psychedelic effects after swallowing the drug. This was discovered many centuries ago by tribes in the Amazon. They mixed the DMT-containing *Psychotria viridis* with a climbing vine that contains these inhibitors – *B. caapi* – and called the resulting brew 'ayahuasca'.

Having said it is natural, the DMT found outside the Amazon is just as likely to be synthesised as it is to be extracted from plants, so it might not be quite as natural as some people would like to believe. DMT in the UK is usually found as a white or yellow crystalline powder or solid lump.

What are the short-term effects?

The effects of DMT will depend on the method of consumption. When DMT powder is snorted, smoked or injected the entire intoxication experience will usually last less than an hour. However, when ayahuasca is consumed orally, the intoxication experience will take longer to begin, usually half an hour or more, and can last for four or even up to ten hours.

The psychedelic trip on DMT is largely similar to that experienced on LSD or psilocybin – perceptual alterations are common, distortions of time, vivid colours, visions or hallucinations, and some people even report feelings of communing with other worlds, and other beings.

As well as the psychedelic effects, DMT, and particularly ayahuasca may induce nausea and vomiting, euphemistically referred to as 'purging' in some ayahuasca ceremonies, and stomach cramps.

What are the longer-term effects?

Similarly to LSD and psilocybin, there do not seem to be many long-term risks from taking DMT. Much like other psychedelics, if a person has a predisposition to poor mental health, for example family history of psychosis or schizophrenia, then DMT could exacerbate this or potentially even trigger an episode of poor mental health. As such, people who are worried about their mental health should not take psychedelics without guidance from a medical professional.

As with LSD and psilocybin, tolerance to DMT builds up extremely quickly – if you attempt to use DMT twice in quick succession, you will not experience intoxication the second time. Users report that they wait between trips in order for this tolerance to diminish.

Myths and misconceptions

DMT doesn't affect the brain, it affects the soul

Whether a psychedelic experience like DMT affects the soul or not is perhaps not a matter for science. Some people may believe that their soul or something integral to their 'self' is altered after taking a substance. However, given the high molecular similarity between DMT and the neurotransmitter serotonin, and what we know about the brain from animal and neurocognitive research, it is safe to say that DMT affects the brain.

? PROBABLY UNTRUE

The pineal gland produces DMT at extraordinary moments in our lives

Something that has puzzled researchers for many decades was the discovery in the 1960s of trace levels of DMT in various fluids throughout the human body. This very strongly suggests that, much like with cannabis and morphine, our bodies make endogenous DMT. However, as yet nobody has been able to prove with any certainty what the purpose of endogenous DMT is.

Rick Strassman is a clinical associate professor of psychiatry in the USA, and has researched and written a book about DMT. Strassman believes DMT is produced during dreaming, and in the moments before death. However, there's very little evidence for this. As for it being made in the pineal gland – again this is unclear. Recently researchers found trace amounts of DMT in rat pineal glands, but this hasn't been replicated in humans.

At a recent conference, researcher Dr David Nichols pointed out that the amounts of endogenous DMT found in humans are at levels far too low to induce a meaningful psychedelic effect – he suggested it would be perfectly plausible that the DMT found in humans could be a by-product – given how similar DMT is to well-established neurotransmitters like serotonin and tryptophan.

Of course, not knowing doesn't mean that Strassman isn't right. Maybe the pineal gland is some sort of 'third eye' or 'seat of the soul', and DMT floods forth while we're asleep, or as we are about to pass away. However, given how much we know about other neurotransmitters, and about other functions of the pineal gland, I'm a little sceptical to be honest with you.

? PROBABLY MYTH

Are the different tryptamine psychedelics related to different types of psychedelic experience?

If you ask a person who uses psychedelics to talk about their trip experiences, they will often tell you that the type of intoxication experience they have on LSD is markedly different compared to mushrooms, above and beyond the length and the intensity of a trip. People who use DMT are far more likely to report 'meeting' or conversing with beings of some kind, compared to people using LSD or mushrooms. But understanding why this might be is incredibly difficult.

As is apparent throughout this book, the set and setting in which you take a drug – and the expectations you have about its effect – are hugely important in defining the experience that you will have. This is never truer than for psychedelics, where the experience is so personal and subjective.

In his book *DMT: The Spirit Molecule*, Rick Strassman invites the reader to ponder the language used to describe a psychedelic drug, the person consuming it, and the person administering it. Are you a celebrant, taking a sacrament from a shaman? Are you a psychonaut using an illicit drug to expand your mind? Or are you a research participant being given a medication to induce a psychotic-like experience from a doctor? Do you think this would impact your expectations of how the substance would affect you?

It is incredibly difficult to tease all this apart. And as such, it's hard to know whether certain trip experiences appearing more with one particular psychedelic (such as seeing figures when taking DMT) are because a person is expecting these to happen, where this isn't the case for psilocybin or LSD.

The types of visions or experiences people have during psychedelic trips certainly seem to be influenced by things like culture – it looks as if the drugs are working with what's already in your mind, rather than creating something completely new. But as to whether they really induce different experiences – that's much harder to investigate.

If you're considering taking part in an ayahuasca ritual, it is important to note that the brew you will drink can have harmful interactions with certain other drugs, including antidepressants such as selective-serotonin reuptake inhibitors (SSRIs) and benzodiazepines such as diazepam or alprazolam (Xanax).

Focus on: Depressants

Depressants, or 'downers', are substances that will lower levels of arousal. By that I don't mean sexual arousal (some of these drugs have quite the opposite effect where that is concerned), but I mean the general functioning of brain and body.

People use downers for many reasons. For some, they can lower inhibitions and make socialising more fun. For others, they can aid with relaxation, potentially being used to help someone get to sleep, or to block out or numb painful thoughts or memories. Some might turn to these drugs to manage chronic pain symptoms, or anxiety, or even difficult life circumstances. The reasons people have for taking these substances can impact on how likely they are to develop dependence from using them.

Which drugs are depressants?

Drugs that are classed as depressants or 'downers' include opioids (such as heroin or prescription opioids), benzodiazepines, and anaesthetics like nitrous oxide and ketamine. Some drugs can be hard to categorise – a number of depressants have paradoxical stimulant-like effects at low doses. Alcohol and kratom are two such substances. GHB is a depressant.

What effects do depressants have?

As the name suggests, depressants will depress some of the functions of the body. This could mean breathing, which might become slower or shallower after consuming some of these substances, or heart rate, which can slow. It could also mean cognitive abilities – it might become harder to think or perform complicated mental tasks after consuming these substances. Reaction times can also be slowed, which is why driving or operating heavy machinery is particularly dangerous while intoxicated (though this is true for almost all psychoactive drugs).

In some cases, the ability to move around at all might become substantially impaired – a number of these substances are prescribed as sedatives or anaesthetics, designed to keep people still, calm, and pain free.

At high doses, depressants can be dangerous, as they can slow the body and brain to the point of loss of consciousness. At this point, people are in danger of choking if they vomit, or being taken advantage of, robbed or assaulted, while unable to look after themselves. If breathing or heart rate continue to drop, then the person is at very real risk of coma or death, and should be taken to a hospital as soon as possible.

Interactions

Mixing depressants with other depressants is dangerous – their combined effects on breathing or heart rate could dramatically increase the chance of coma or death. There's also increased risk from using depressants and stimulants together, as they can mask the effects of each other and lead to an individual taking higher doses of both, putting themselves in more danger of overdose, increasing the chance of tolerance or dependence, and putting more strain on their body.

CHAPTER 9

E-cigarettes

NICOTINE

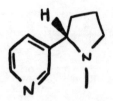

What is it? A method of consuming nicotine that doesn't involve burning tobacco, instead nicotine solution is heated and the vapour inhaled.

Type of drug: Nicotine is a stimulant.

Popularity: Mostly used among people who are trying to give up cigarettes. There is worry in the USA that use is growing among children and young people, but rates are still low.

How consumed: Vaping.

Timescale: Slightly slower nicotine absorption compared to smoking cigarettes.

Some effects: Similar to cigarettes.

I THOUGHT LONG and hard about whether to do a single chapter about nicotine, the psychoactive substance found in tobacco products and e-cigarettes. In the end I decided to separate out tobacco and e-cigarettes, because e-cigarettes regularly make the news across the world, are treated very differently in different parts of the world, and have a load of myths and misconceptions about them that are quite separate from those that exist around tobacco products.

E-cigarettes, or devices containing nicotine, are banned in some countries like Australia, and completely unregulated in others. Some people think they are every bit as dangerous as cigarettes, while others believe they could be a hugely important harm-reduction device to help smokers stop using cigarettes.

What is it?

First off – what are e-cigarettes, also known as vapes or vaping pens? There are a number of different types of vaping device available, but all are devices that allow the inhalation of a vapour that usually (but not always) contains nicotine. The main constituent of e-cigarette liquid is usually propylene glycol (also known as E1520, an additive used in food preparation), or glycerine, a by-product of soap manufacture that is made from either animal or vegetable fat. Some e-cigarette liquids will also contain flavourings, which can be made from a number of different chemicals depending on the type of flavour (more on that later).

All the devices work by using a battery to heat up a metal element that turns the e-liquid into a vapour, which can then be inhaled by the user. So actually, e-cigarettes are neither electronic, nor cigarettes. Confusing, huh?

As for the different types – when e-cigarettes first appeared on the market, in the early to mid-2000s, they tended to look somewhat like oversized cigarettes. Their LED tips glowed red (or sometimes blue) when you took a drag on them, mimicking a real cigarette. But this is really where the similarities ended. These types of device, known as first-generation e-cigarettes or 'cigalikes', were not very efficient at delivering nicotine. Second-generation e-cigarettes are the devices that look like sonic screwdrivers, or fountain pens for those not as *au fait* with *Doctor Who* as me.

Where first-generation cigalikes were disposable, or had disposable cartridges containing the fluid, these second-generation devices were refillable, meaning you could buy liquid and top it up yourself. Do you want lemon-meringue-pie vape, or blue-raspberry? These were the first devices where flavourings became more commonly used. They were better at delivering nicotine, but still fell substantially short of the nicotine 'hit' smokers experience from cigarettes.

Third-generation devices were much more malleable. They are often known as 'mods' due to their modular properties, and with these devices it's possible to manipulate the voltage as well as the liquid, which can impact on nicotine delivery. More recently still, devices that use nicotine salts have begun to be marketed (one device in particular, called Juul, is hugely popular in the USA). These fourth-generation devices look like USB sticks – they're small and discreet – and the nicotine liquid is contained in disposable pods, rather than being refillable.

The first e-cigarette was invented by Chinese pharmacist Hon Lik in Beijing in 2003. It is reported that he was looking for a way of helping himself to quit smoking after his father, who was also a heavy smoker, died of lung cancer. We know a lot about how and why tobacco, and in particular cigarettes, are bad for us, and we also know that it can be extremely difficult for some people to give up smoking.

Nicotine-replacement therapy can be effective for some people, but these gums, patches or nasal sprays cannot deliver nicotine with anything like the spike that a cigarette can – nicotine absorbed through the skin or the lining of the mouth or nose takes substantially longer to get into the bloodstream than it does from a cigarette, where the smoke is drawn into the lungs and absorbed into the blood within seconds.

E-cigarettes are appealing to smokers who are trying to stop or cut down their smoking, as they can deliver nicotine in a slightly more effective way than other nicotine-replacement therapy. The e-cigarette user will not get yellow-stained fingers, or bad breath that can be a result of smoking cigarettes.

A person is also likely to be putting themselves at vastly reduced risk of cancers and lung disease if they can switch from smoking to using an e-cigarette, as there is no tobacco being burnt in an e-cigarette – the nicotine contained is heated up but not burnt, and tobacco is not present at all. Crucially, this also means there is no tar. Public Health England published a report of e-cigarette research in 2015 where they estimated that e-cigarettes are up to 95-per-cent less harmful than smoking (more on this later).

But are e-cigarettes appealing to anyone else? A number of individuals who work in public health, in the UK but particularly in the USA, Canada and Australia, are concerned that e-cigarettes might also be appealing to young people, even children. Tobacco smoking rates have been falling consistently, year on year, for many decades now, particularly among young people. Could e-cigarettes reverse that trend, or get a generation previously uninterested in tobacco newly dependent on nicotine?

At the moment, this worry seems to be unfounded, certainly in the UK. Many surveys are conducted each year to monitor the use of e-cigarettes among young people. In the UK the use of these devices by eleven- to eighteen-year-olds is increasing slightly year on year, but regular use remains very low.

A 2018 survey conducted by YouGov and Action on Smoking and Health (ASH) found that while roughly a third of young people might have experimented with them recently, only 2 per cent of those surveyed report using e-cigarettes weekly, and over three-quarters of those asked have never tried one at all. Only 5 per cent of young people who reported never smoking a tobacco cigarette had ever tried an e-cigarette, with less than 1 per cent using them regularly.

However, this pattern isn't necessarily the same as in other places around the world – as different countries have differing legislation around e-cigarettes, and alternative products available on the market. In the USA, for example, there are no limits to the concentration of nicotine within e-liquid, as there are in countries within the European Union. In the last year or two, researchers have noticed that the patterns of youth use between the UK and the USA are diverging – with eighteen-year-olds in America increasingly reporting having at the very least experimented with vaping.

There are a number of theories as to why this might be. One thought is the types of device available: in the USA, Juul-brand devices are extremely popular among young people. As I described earlier, these devices look like USB sticks, come in a range of colours, and deliver nicotine in an extremely effective way, as they contain nicotine salts rather than freebase nicotine (see below), which for various chemical reasons means nicotine can be inhaled at higher levels without it feeling as harsh on the throat.

While Juul products are available in the UK, the strength of nicotine is limited by EU regulations, meaning it is often lower than levels found in the USA. This difference could also be due to the way the question is asked in various surveys. In the UK, surveys often focus on regular or recent use, while in the USA young people have been asked whether they have ever tried e-cigarettes. It's easy to see why this could lead to a situation where it appears that e-cigs are much more common in the USA. Either way, it's something that researchers on both sides of the Atlantic will be keeping an eye on.

What are the short-term effects?

As with tobacco cigarettes, the short-term 'intoxication' effects of e-cigarettes are due to the nicotine present in e-liquid. Nicotine is a mild stimulant, so will have the short-term effects all stimulants have – it will raise a person's heart rate and blood pressure, and it might make an individual feel slightly more alert or awake.

As mentioned earlier, e-cigarettes are not as effective at delivering nicotine as tobacco cigarettes, but they are getting better – in particular the devices that use nicotine salts rather than freebase nicotine (freebase is how nicotine is usually encountered, for example in e-liquid. A salt in this context is a freebase compound mixed with an acid).

What are the longer-term effects?

It is the longer-term impacts of e-cigarettes that are more up for debate at present. The devices have not been around for very long, in research terms; only a couple of decades. We know that they don't contain many of the compounds in tobacco smoke that cause a lot of the harms we know about from smoking. We know that they do contain some of these other chemicals, but at orders of magnitude lower than seen in tobacco smoke.

So far, a lot of the evidence about the harms from e-cigarette vapour has come from cell culture studies. A number of these studies have suggested substantial harm to cell cultures from e-cigarette vapour being passed across them. However, it's important to note that where these harms are then compared to the harms from having tobacco smoke passed across them, the harms are substantially greater from tobacco smoke.

All this isn't to say that there aren't any risks from using e-cigarettes, and of course it's possible that there are other threats – different from smoking – that we don't know about yet. Time, and research, will tell. As I said earlier, there's been a rather confusing statement made by Public Health England, a government-funded body in the UK who have synthesised evidence around the devices, that e-cigarettes are 95-per-cent safer than tobacco cigarettes. This statement is likely quite accurate, but also quite hard to interpret.

Firstly, 95-per-cent safer than smoking doesn't mean 95-per-cent safe – this is a relative risk rather than an absolute risk. Smoking is one of the most uniquely harmful activities a person can do – so something with a reduced risk in comparison to smoking could still be quite harmful. The purpose of presenting this figure in this way is to encourage those who currently smoke to consider switching to something far less harmful that could still satiate their desire for nicotine. It's not to say that vaping is safe, harmless, or without risk. But if you're a regular smoker, vaping is clearly safer than continuing to smoke.

Some people who use e-cigarettes will not quit smoking, and will use both cigarettes and e-cigarettes, potentially for many years. People using e-cigarettes in this way, potentially to cut down but not completely stop using cigarettes, might believe that they would experience health benefits from doing so. However, at the moment the little evidence available suggests this is not the case.

A study compared people using various different combinations of cigarette, e-cigarette, and nicotine-replacement therapy (NRT) use over a prolonged period of time. They found similar levels of nicotine across all groups in the study. When looking at exposure to carcinogens and toxicants, though, they found lower levels for people using only NRT, or only e-cigarettes, compared to cigarettes. For individuals dual-using, the levels of carcinogens and toxicants were no different to people who were just using cigarettes.

These results are from only one study, and could indicate

differences in heaviness of smoking prior to the start of the study, for example, but they might suggest that in order to experience health benefits from using e-cigarettes, a person must stop smoking completely. And how easy is that?

Does taking up vaping actually help people to give up tobacco cigarettes? There are a number of large-scale trials going on to investigate this topic, and at present the evidence suggests 'probably yes'. However, there are disagreements within the literature, largely dependent on how these clinical trials were set up to investigate it.

Myths and misconceptions

Nicotine causes cancer and nicotine is still in e-cigarettes

Smoking cigarettes hugely increases your risk of lung cancer, and indeed a number of other cancers including breast cancer, mouth cancer, liver cancer, colon cancer and many others. But contrary to popular belief, it's not the nicotine in cigarettes that causes this huge increase. There's no evidence that nicotine causes cancer in humans. There is some evidence from rodent studies that nicotine, without the other constituents of tobacco, can cause tumours.

As yet this hasn't been found in humans, and while there is some disagreement about whether nicotine might indirectly increase the risk of cancer, all researchers agree that this likelihood is far smaller than the risk from smoking cigarettes.

? PROBABLY MYTH

E-cigarettes encourage young people to start smoking – and nicotine harms their developing brains

E-cigarettes might be effective to help people quit smoking – but what if they also have the opposite effect, and encourage some young people to take up smoking? E-cigarettes still for the most part contain nicotine, which is the substance that can lead to dependence on cigarettes. What if young people experiment with these devices and become dependent on nicotine, then turn to cigarettes to deliver nicotine in a more effective way?

While this is a possibility, and something researchers are actively monitoring, as yet there is no evidence that this is the case. Smoking rates across the world are going down, and there doesn't seem to be any sign of this trend reversing since e-cigarettes have appeared. And this decline is true even when you look only at the data in young people – removing those older individuals who may have used e-cigarettes to help them quit smoking.

Some researchers, particularly those in the USA, have argued that nicotine is harmful to the developing brain, and as such youth e-cigarette use should be a cause for concern in and of itself. At the moment, pretty much all the evidence for this comes from rodent studies, rather than humans. Rodents given nicotine during their 'adolescence' show more impulsive behaviours as adults than their non-exposed counterparts. But whether this would also happen in humans is not known.

? UNCLEAR/PARTLY UNTRUE

E-cigarettes cause 'popcorn lung' – bronchiolitis obliterans

This myth came about because a study analysed a number of e-liquid samples in the USA, and found that some e-cigarette liquids contained a buttery food flavouring called diacetyl. This chemical is used in popcorn making (it's approved safe to eat, but tests didn't assess risks from inhalation), and became linked to bronchiolitis obliterans in 2002, when a research article reported about eight cases of the disease at a popcorn factory over a period of eight years. However, the paper itself was somewhat inconclusive about whether diacetyl was a causal factor in these cases.

Since 2016, the UK requires that e-liquids do not contain diacetyl, so the somewhat tenuous link between e-cigarettes and popcorn lung doesn't exist anymore, certainly not in the UK anyway. It is also worth highlighting that to date there have been no reported cases of popcorn lung in people who use e-cigarettes, and that diacetyl is also found, and at far higher levels, in tobacco cigarette smoke. Yet you never hear that smoking will cause popcorn lung.

 MYTH

OK, but vaping causes pneumonia, right?

Headlines in the UK press in early 2018 suggested that e-cigarettes might increase the risk of pneumonia. These were based on a research paper that investigated whether using an e-cigarette increases the number of pneumococcal bacteria sticking to the cells in a person's airways, though it didn't measure this directly. Whether this increased sticking substantially increases the risk of pneumonia is also less than clear, so concluding that vaping causes pneumonia is incorrect from this evidence.

There has been further research published that has found evidence of bacteria and fungi in e-liquids. This research was conducted in the USA, and it's worth pointing out that there are tighter restrictions on both devices and liquid production in Europe than in the USA. As is always the case, the better quality the product, the less risk of corners being cut in the manufacturing process and impurities creeping in. Where e-cigarettes are concerned, it is better to buy regulated products than knock-offs that won't have been subject to regulation and checks.

There is a far rarer type of pneumonia called lipoid or lipid pneumonia that is caused by fat being inhaled into the lungs.

There have been a few case reports published in medical journals of e-cigarette users developing this condition, which have concluded that the condition might have been due to the fatty glycerine used in e-liquid somehow getting into an individual's lungs. However, these cases are extremely rare – they could conceivably be due to incorrect usage or a faulty device.

The most common causes of lipoid pneumonia are people accidentally inhaling olive oil, milk or egg-yolks, oil-based medication or nasal drops, or oils such as WD-40, paints or lubricants. It's also occasionally seen in people who 'eat fire', if they accidentally inhale kerdan, a type of petroleum used in fire-breathing performances.

? PARTLY TRUE

E-cigarettes are dangerous – they explode and injure people or start fires

Cases of e-cigarettes exploding make grisly headlines. They have been implicated in a few hundred fires in the UK over the past few years. In almost all of these cases this is where people have used generic or different chargers than the charger provided with the device, or where the e-cigarette or charger has been damaged. The risk of fire is not trivial, but it is also worth remembering that the London Fire Brigade report that the most common cause of fire fatalities is smoking and they endorse switching from smoking to vaping as a way of preventing fires.

In the last five years, there are on average twenty-two fires *every week* linked to smoking, in London alone. Many of these are caused by people falling asleep while holding a lit cigarette – as the London Fire Brigade point out, falling asleep while vaping doesn't pose these risks!

? PARTLY TRUE

E-cigarettes are bad for the environment

A large public health organisation in the USA that promotes a tobacco-free future recently published a blog stating that e-cigarettes (in particular Juul devices) are harming the environment, due to their need for single-use plastics, their disposable nature, and that they contain heavy metals, which are seen as a biohazard. While all of these things are true, the fact is that tobacco cigarettes contain heavy metals and other contaminants at a far higher level. Not only that, but cigarette butts dropped on the ground are a huge environmental problem.

A commentary in the journal *Tobacco Control* has estimated that 5.6 trillion cigarette butts are dropped each year, and account for 25 to 50 per cent of the litter collected from roads and streets. Cigarette butts are also the most commonly found litter on beaches, which is potentially an even greater problem, as contact with water can release the heavy metals they contain into seas or other water bodies, where they can cause harm to plants and animals living there.

? PARTLY TRUE

What don't we know?

As is probably apparent from the rest of this chapter, there's still a lot we don't know about e-cigarettes and about vaping. We still don't know for sure whether there will be any long-term risks from them, and if so to what level. We are still investigating how effective e-cigarettes are to help people stop smoking, and whether e-cigarettes are acting as a gateway drug to smoking for young people, or if and how they are being used by young people more generally. There are new products emerging all the time, and there is a lot of research going on at the moment.

By the time you are reading this, our knowledge of e-cigarettes will hopefully have improved. Will this mean researchers will begin to agree on their risks or potential harm-reduction properties? . . . Well, we will see.

While I was finalising this book, there was a bit of a development around e-cigarettes in the USA. In August, a death that was attributed to e-cigarettes occurred. This was the first death linked to e-cigarettes ever. Since then, there have been reports of further illnesses, and several more deaths, mostly among men. As yet, the reasons for these deaths are not clear. There haven't been any reported outside the USA, and the majority of those investigated have been linked to the vaping of cannabinoids, rather than nicotine. There's some suggestion that this could be related to the use of illicit THC vape liquid containing substances that are used in topical and oral preparations of THC, but that when heated by an e-cigarette could become toxic: in particular vitamin E acetate has been implicated. But at the moment it's unclear. As I write this, we don't know what has caused these deaths, and of course an outbreak of unexplained deaths is extremely worrying. However, that these deaths are only occurring in one country, and not anywhere else, does hint that it is unlikely to be e-cigarettes themselves, but some substance or adulterant specific to use in the USA, that might be causing this. Different organisations have reacted very differently to these deaths – some US based organisations have suggested that e-cigarettes should all be completely banned. Others are being more measured and advising that people should only use regulated products (this is always extremely good advice), because there is a far greater risk of illness and death from smoking tobacco than using e-cigarettes. It can be incredibly hard to tease out what we know from the hyperbole that surrounds e-cigs, but we know that if you're trying to quit smoking, it's better to use an e-cig than to smoke cigarettes. But stick to the regulated products.

CHAPTER 10

GHB

What is it? Synthetic substance found in liquid or powder form.
Type of drug: Depressant.
Popularity: Unclear, as not much data collected, although what
is available suggests it's not overly common, even among
people who use other drugs.
How consumed: Usually mixed into a liquid (not alcohol) and
drunk.
Some effects: Euphoria, relaxation, disorientation, drowsiness.

THE PRESS IN the UK refer to it as 'liquid ecstasy', and it has
been linked to date rapes, club culture, gay culture and body-
building. More recently it is being portrayed as a drug popular
with young women who want to go out dancing, who might be
concerned about the calories contained in alcohol and are looking
for a substance with a similar intoxication effect without the
sugar content. But headlines in the press also warn of its ability
to melt plastic, and the high risk of overdose from use of it.

What is it?

GHB, or to give it its chemical name Gamma-hydroxybutyric acid, is a depressant, made in small quantities by the human body. Closely related to GHB are GBL (Gamma-butyrolactone) and 1,4-Butanediol – GHB 'prodrugs' or precursors that the body converts into GHB when they are consumed. All these substances are usually encountered in a powder or colourless and odourless liquid form, which can be added to beverages and drunk.

While GHB is often a controlled substance, GBL and 1,4-BD are found in some cleaning products, meaning they are potentially easier to get hold of. In Australia, GHB is often referred to as G, or Juice.

What are the short-term effects?

Many people who use GHB report doing so because of its similarity, in terms of intoxication effect, to alcohol. If a person takes GHB, they will experience onset of intoxication within about fifteen minutes, and this will then last for a couple of hours. GHB can make people feel chilled out, make them feel euphoric, and some people report feeling sexually aroused or horny when intoxicated. However, although it's thought of as a sex drug, intoxication on GHB can also make it harder for men to ejaculate.

Similarly to alcohol, GHB can lower inhibition, which can lead to an increased risk of partaking in unsafe sex, and because of that an increased possibility of contracting an STD, or even of having sex with someone you wouldn't normally have sex with.

At higher doses, GHB can make a person feel dizzy or confused. It can increase feelings of disorientation, and can make people feel drowsy. It's not uncommon for people using GHB for the first time to vomit, and high doses can also induce vomiting, much like alcohol. GHB can cause stiffening of the muscles, which can make movement harder. People report twitching, dribbling and finding themselves unable to sit or stand up straight. At higher doses still, GHB can cause people to pass out, and can induce respiratory collapse. At these levels there is the risk of seizures, coma and even death.

When people are having a night out and using GHB multiple times, there are further dangers. Due to the impact of GHB on short-term memory, it's easy to forget how much you have taken, and when. As such, people will often set themselves reminders on their smartphones, so they know not to take any more GHB for at least a couple of hours. Anecdotal evidence also suggests that the more doses a person consumes on a particular evening or session, the higher the chances of them passing out or experiencing bad effects from doing so, although this is possibly due to the increased likelihood to misjudge either the individual dose, or the time between doses.

GHB is a particularly dangerous substance to take when you are alone – in case you need an ambulance or help after an accidental overdose. People who regularly use GHB report that losing consciousness, while not being something they ever intend to do, does happen, and when it does they are reliant on friends taking care of them. Should you find yourself in this situation with someone who has passed out, the advice is to put them in the recovery position on their side, and keep checking their breathing – if it slows, call an ambulance immediately.

What is it about GHB that is particularly risky in this regard? As well as it impacting on memory and judgment, maybe making intoxicated people more likely to take a dose sooner than they should, the doses involved are extremely small, which is problematic for a couple of reasons. If a person is using a syringe* to measure their dose, this might get harder as they get more intoxicated throughout the evening, meaning errors are more likely. Because the dose is so small, a small increase could have big consequences.

More perilous still, GHB has what is known as a small window of efficacy. By this I mean that there is only a very small difference in dose between an amount that will give the effect a person desires, and the amount that will push them into toxicity, and lead to extremely negative effects. This problem is compounded by the illicit nature of the substance – it's likely that different batches of GHB will be differing strengths, meaning that a dose from one batch, despite being the same volume of liquid, could be far stronger, and therefore extremely dangerous.

It's really hazardous to add these substances to alcohol, as the depressant effects of each will be emphasised and the risks from consuming too much are therefore higher. Not only that, but because the dosage is very small, when people administer it into their drinks using a syringe, a difference of millilitres can impact whether the dose is enjoyable or enough to induce unconsciousness. And GHB and GBL have different dosing, so this can also be problematic for people using the substance. There are other analogues of GHB too, including substances like 1,4-Butanediol, which also have different dosages and can lead to dangers.

Much like many other substances in this book, GHB is particularly risky to people who have underlying health problems related to their blood pressure, either high or low. It's also thought to be unsafe for people who have epilepsy or a history of convulsions, and to people with pre-existing heart or breathing problems. GHB is also harmful if consumed neat, rather than mixed into

---

* People will often put a pen mark on a syringe, so they know where to fill the syringe up to – however, GHB can dissolve the ink, often resulting in the pen mark becoming faded or disappearing over time, possibly as intoxication is increasing, too. A bad combo.

a drink. It can cause damage to the mouth, teeth, throat and stomach if consumed in this way.

What are the longer-term effects?

Longer term, there's some suggestion that people become tolerant to GHB, needing higher doses to get the same effect. There is also growing evidence that GHB can lead to psychological and physical dependence. Warning signs for dependence can include motivation or reasons for using. If individuals are using GHB 'to cope', for example to manage symptoms of trauma or poor mental health, to aid with sleeping, or to numb painful feelings, or are using it alone rather than in social settings – this may be an indicator that a person is becoming reliant on it.

Clinics that work with individuals dependent on GHB see some people who are using the substance multiple times throughout the day, and even waking up during the night to take GHB in order to avoid withdrawal symptoms. Those people trying to stop using the substance report withdrawal symptoms that include delirium, psychosis, tremors, insomnia and severe anxiety. Due to this, it is strongly advised that individuals who want to stop using it should seek medical support to do so.

Trying to reduce or stop using GHB without medical support is extremely risky, as seizures can also occur as part of withdrawal, and individuals may need hospitalisation for treatment. Withdrawals can be particularly complex if individuals are using GHB in combination with other substances (more on that later).

Myths and misconceptions

GHB is a gay drug

GHB has a reputation in the media for being a drug used particularly by homosexual men, as a club drug, a chillout substance and something used during sex to enhance the experience. Actually, there have been very few large-scale surveys of who uses GHB, so this may not present the whole picture.

The Global Drugs Survey, which takes place every year, uses opportunistic sampling – they ask people to take part, and to share the survey among their friends, rather than trying to recruit a random and therefore representative sample. As such, it is not a good way to work out what is the prevalence of use of a substance in the general population, as people are far more likely to fill it in if they use drugs than if they don't, because of the nature of the survey. However, it can give a good indication of how commonly used a particular substance is among people who use drugs in general, and it can also give an idea of what groups of people might be particularly likely to use a particular substance.

In their 2018 report, the Global Drugs Survey noted that use of GHB is low, even among a sample of individuals where drug use is over-represented. They reported that GHB was used by 1.4 per cent of straight men who filled in their survey, 4.4 per cent of homosexual* men, 0.8 per cent of straight women and 1.9 per cent of gay or bisexual women in the previous year. However, while this might look like it's predominantly used by gay men, the number of people in each of those groups is important.

They point out that there are more straight men than gay men who filled out the survey, and as such, in absolute numbers the largest group reporting using GHB were straight men. Not only

---

* They don't report about bisexual men for some reason – presumably they are included in this category as is the case for women.

that, but their report also found that those gay men who were using GHB were doing so infrequently (roughly sixteen times a year), which led them to conclude 'the stereotype of dependent users is also challenged'.

However, other research suggests dependence on GHB might be on the rise – certainly in Australia, where research is taking place. Addiction researcher Dr Shalini Arunogiri works with individuals who use GHB in Melbourne, Australia. She told me she is seeing an increase in dependent users where she works, and that this pattern is also being seen in the UK and across Europe.

Other studies have found that despite its reputation as a club drug, GHB is most commonly consumed in private residences rather than in these settings. This might suggest that rather than a club drug, it's a post-club drug. But in reality, we know very little about who is using GHB, and how, and also very little about who is likely to develop problems or experience harms from doing so.

✗ MYTH

GHB is a sex-attack drug

There have been cases where GHB has been implicated as a date-rape drug. The substance can make an individual feel out of it, and even fall unconscious, and it has been linked to sexual assault and rape of both women and men. However, while being vigilant with your drink when you're out is always a good idea, is there any truth to GHB being used in this way?

A 2006 study by the Association of Chief Police Officers suggests maybe not. They found that of 120 instances of alleged drug-facilitated sexual assaults, in only two cases was GHB found to be the substance used. A systematic review on this topic was conducted in 2010. The authors of this research found very few studies that had assessed the use of GHB in drug-facilitated sexual assaults of women. In what few studies they identified, they found rates of positive screening for GHB at around 4 per cent in the USA, less than 1 per cent in the UK, and a similar rate in France – the only three locations where data was available.

However, they also point out that screening for GHB in these cases had only been introduced relatively recently. Not only that, but given the large percentage of sexual assaults that go unreported, and the short half-life of GHB in the body meaning a delay in screening might miss its use, they suggest true rates might be higher than their results indicate.

GHB is also naturally found in low levels in the human body – in various different bodily fluids and tissues, including blood and urine. It's not really clear why, but GHB appears to be related to the naturally occurring neurotransmitter GABA. This presence of naturally occurring GHB can make it even more challenging for police to determine whether low levels of GHB found are due to a drink being spiked, or simply naturally occurring GHB produced within the body.

? PARTLY TRUE

GHB helps bodybuilders bulk up

Research into GHB has noted that it increases slow-wave sleep (as opposed to REM sleep). During slow-wave sleep, a growth hormone is secreted into the body. Because of this, GHB was popular with bodybuilders during the 1990s and more recently as they believed it could help them bulk up. However, the evidence that GHB actually leads to measureable differences in body mass is extremely thin on the ground, and some experts suggest that levels of growth hormone might only increase for very brief amounts of time after taking it, meaning it's probably not a sensible strategy to employ for individuals looking to gain muscle.

? PROBABLY MYTH

Does GHB have any medical uses?

GHB is available as a medication in the USA, although it is rarely prescribed. In the past, it was used as a pre-medication to help patients sleep prior to surgery. It is also prescribed for the treatment of narcolepsy – a rare condition where the brain is unable to regulate sleep patterns, meaning people can fall asleep at inappropriate moments.

GHB is the active compound in the branded medication Xyrem, which is prescribed for cataplexy (sudden weakness in muscles caused by strong emotion such as laughter, anger or surprise), and what's termed 'excessive daytime sleepiness'. There is also some history of GHB being used to help people undergoing withdrawal from dependent alcohol use, although there are more effective medications for this, so it's rarely used in this way.

Although not recognised as a treatment, GHB is also very occasionally prescribed 'off-label' for the treatment of fibromy-algia, a poorly understood condition that causes pain throughout the body, and a heightened pain response.

GHB and other drugs

I've already mentioned that GHB is particularly risky if mixed with alcohol. Unfortunately, co-use with alcohol is common as the drug is taken where people are socialising, which often goes hand in hand with alcohol consumption. But GHB is also more dangerous if co-used with stimulants. Some people might use a stimulant such as amphetamine, cocaine, or even a caffeinated energy drink, in order to stay awake for longer while intoxicated on GHB. But stimulants can mask the effects of GHB, which can then result in accidental overdose, as the margins of too-little to too-much for GHB are so small.

Some individuals use GHB to manage the comedown or withdrawal from stimulants such as methamphetamine. This co-use is risky as dependence can then form to both substances. Not only that, but treatment clinics report that withdrawal from GHB can be more complicated and unpleasant – not to mention dangerous – where individuals are also using stimulants like methamphetamine.

CHAPTER 11

Heroin

What is it? Semi-synthetic substance derived from opium extracted from poppies.

Type of drug: Opioid depressant.

Popularity: Not one of the most popular psychoactive substances, but with a disproportionate number of deaths from using as the risk of overdose is high, and can be fatal.

How consumed: Usually smoked or injected.

Some effects: Rush of euphoria, pain relief, relaxation, nausea, slower and shallower breathing, weakened pulse.

WHEN I WAS growing up in the 1980s and 1990s, heroin was portrayed in the media as the demon drug. A drug that was linked to the most terrifying illness of the time: AIDS. A drug that seemed to lead to addiction in almost everyone who used it. *Trainspotting* was the first film I ever watched in surround sound (an odd choice, I know). It didn't shy away from portraying the risks of injecting, or the lifestyle and environmental factors that might lead someone towards starting to use heroin, and developing a problem with it.

But how realistic was its – and my – perception of the drug? Is one use really all it takes to develop a habit?

What is it?

To start with the basics, heroin is the street name for the compound diamorphine. It is semi-synthetic – opium from poppies is chemically processed to make it stronger (stronger meaning a lower dose is needed to get the same effect, not that the intoxication effect itself is stronger, an important distinction). Heroin produced in different regions of the world can have different appearances. Sometimes it can be found as a white or brown powder, while it can also be encountered as a thick solid known as 'black tar' heroin.

Heroin is an opioid – the name used to refer to substances derived from opium poppies. Technically, opioids are substances where some chemical alteration has been made to the opium (so synthetic or semi-synthetic substances), whereas substances like morphine and codeine that can be extracted directly from opium are known as opiates (having said this, these terms are now often used interchangeably).

Interestingly, humans also have a number of endogenous opioids – that is, compounds similar to opium from poppies are made by our bodies. There are a few of these – one is endorphin, the chemical our brain releases to inhibit pain and induce euphoria. We have opioid receptors in our brain and nervous system because of these endogenous opioids, and it's at these sites that external opioids and opiates can have their effect.

Heroin can be consumed in a number of ways. The powder can be 'smoked' (I use inverted commas because smoking suggests burning, but really the powder is heated and the vapour inhaled;

it's more like vaping than smoking). If you've heard someone talk about 'chasing the dragon', this is what they're referring to. Heroin powder is placed usually in foil and heated from below, and a tube can be used to inhale the vapour.

Heroin can also be injected. In this instance the powder needs to be combined with an acid of some kind, to create diamorphine hydrochloride. This can then be injected into the bloodstream, either directly into a vein, or under the skin or into a muscle. It's also possible to snort heroin, although this method of consumption is less common. Heroin can also be 'plugged' rectally. This is where it's put in a syringe without the needle on the end, and pushed into the anus. Women can also consume it vaginally.

As with other substances, the method by which you consume it impacts on the intoxication effects. Injecting into the blood-stream is the most 'efficient' way of consuming a drug, if by efficient you mean faster acting. Injected heroin can cross the blood–brain barrier within seconds. Inhaling the vapour is a little slower, but still a pretty quick route to intoxication.

What are the short-term effects?

The initial intoxication experience is often described as a rush of euphoria. How intense this rush is will depend on a number of things, including the method of administration. If heroin is injected into a vein, this will be intense and almost immediate. The effect will be diminished if injected into a muscle or under the skin (subcutaneously). If consumed via snorting, it'll be still less immediate and intense.

Heroin is a sedative, so it will make a person feel peaceful and relaxed. However, it can also cause nausea or vomiting, particu-larly in those who are not experienced users. This is similar to morphine: some people given morphine in a medical setting will find it makes them feel really sick. The combination of sedative effect and risk of vomiting can be dangerous too, increasing the risk of choking on vomit while passed out. Heroin can also cause constipation.

Take too much heroin and overdose risks are extremely dangerous. Heroin will suppress breathing (sometimes called respiratory depression), which can become shallow or even stop. Your pupils will shrink, your extremities and lips can go blue. You might have seizures or start shaking. Your pulse will weaken. Overdose can be fatal.* And this is before we talk about the risks from the illegality of heroin.

There are great risks from consuming an illicit drug via injection. Firstly, where do you get your needles? Often this might mean re-using needles, potentially even sharing them. This is a huge risk for the transmission of blood-borne diseases. The most well-known in relation to heroin use is probably HIV (that causes AIDS), but hepatitis B and C are possibly even greater threats, particularly as treatment and prevention of AIDS improves.

Frequent injections can cause collapsed veins, bacterial infections of the skin and soft tissue, and the risk of abscesses and gangrene. In severe cases this can lead to amputations of limbs, or death from septicaemia or bacterial endocarditis. On top of this, as I mentioned earlier, when you inject heroin it needs to be mixed with an acid in order to allow this. If you don't have access to medical-grade acids for this, you might think that using something like lemon juice would be OK. But using lemon juice

---

* Although if countered quickly, it can be reversible. If a substance called naloxone can be administered to a person who has overdosed, this compound will bind to the sites in the brain where heroin binds, and prevent heroin from doing so. It will bring the person out of overdose, and straight into withdrawal, but it could save their life. The UK is currently introducing the provision of naloxone to police forces, and the peers or family of people who use heroin, in a similar way to epi-pens for people with severe allergies, insulin for those with diabetes, or drugs such as midazolam (a benzo) for people with untreatable epilepsy.

in this way has been known to cause fungal infections, including inside the eyeball.

Yikes. So given this risk, why do people take heroin? What's the appeal? The euphoric rush described earlier, for one. The cliché from *Trainspotting* is that it's better than sex. And the analogy might not be too far off – endorphins, our endogenous opioids, are released during sex. And what leads people to continue using? If you become dependent on heroin, then a strong driver for continued use becomes bringing yourself out of heroin withdrawal (more about that later).

What are the longer-term effects?

If you use heroin regularly, there are longer-term risks. If you take heroin daily or near-daily you'll build up a tolerance – you'll no longer get the same rush from the same dose, and you'll need to keep increasing it to get an equivalent high. And the feeling of the rush decreases over time, too. This can mean that soon you'll feel you need heroin to make you feel 'normal', and if you develop dependence, it may feel like you need to use heroin to bring you out of withdrawal, which can be extremely unpleasant.

So what is withdrawal?

It's not nice. It can feel like a heavy flu – and I don't mean like a bad cold, where it's a struggle to function or do daily chores, I mean full-on unable-to-leave-your-bed flu. You can experience heartburn, sleeplessness, depression, anxiety, paranoia, cramps and vomiting. As with lots of other drugs, withdrawal symptoms are the opposite of intoxication effects. Using heroin induces constipation, so as you might then expect, withdrawal can cause diarrhoea. The physical symptoms of withdrawal will pass after around four days, but it'll be a while before you start to feel better – the parallels to flu are many. Breaking the psychological dependence can be even harder.

A further risk from heavy regular heroin use can be that, due to the numbing and sedative effect of the drug, it can be easy to neglect taking care of yourself. This may be why some people who are dependent on heroin can have poor skin, or lose teeth, and are often underweight. It's not a direct biological effect of the drug necessarily, but related to the effect the drug might have on motivation, and indeed related to who might find themselves dependent on heroin.

It's safe to say that heroin dependence can hugely impact on a person's life. But some of the things I heard about heroin when I was a teenager in the 1990s simply aren't backed up by evidence.

Myths and misconceptions

One dose and you'll be hooked

It is impossible to get addicted to a substance, any substance, after one use. It's possible to enjoy it after one try, to be really keen to take it again because the experience was so pleasurable, whether in a hedonistic way or in a way of making your circumstances or situation more bearable for a few hours. But you cannot become dependent on a substance from using it once. And fewer people than you might think actually develop dependence on heroin. According to the American Society of Addiction Medicine (ASAM), around 23 per cent of those who try heroin will develop opioid dependence, suggesting that 77 per cent of those who try it won't.

Other experts have questioned these figures, believing they might underestimate the number of dependent heroin users, because of how they are conducted. General population surveys or household surveys, for example, may underestimate the number of dependent users, as these individuals are at a higher risk of being in prison, or without a fixed address, due to their heroin dependence. If these people are systematically under-represented in these surveys, it would lead to a bias that would suggest heroin was less dependence forming than it truly is.

So what is the real figure? It's hard to say. A small study attempted to account for this bias, and found some evidence that the figure might be closer to 50/50, or even that around 60 per cent of those who try heroin will develop dependence, although their estimate is very uncertain due to assumptions they had to make, and the small sample size. Animal studies also suggest the risk of dependence is higher than the ASAM's estimate, but humans are not rats, so again it's hard to conclude anything definitive.

But whatever way you slice it, there's absolutely no truth in the idea that you only need to try heroin once to become addicted to it.

✗ MYTH

All heroin users are addicted

As we've seen in the previous myth, many people who try heroin will not develop dependence on it. As for people who start using regularly, well, does regular use mean addiction? This really depends on what you mean by 'addiction'. Regular users of heroin will develop tolerance to the drug. They will experience withdrawal if they stop taking it, and so they are likely to be considered dependent. Addiction is often defined as the continuation of a behaviour even when there are real or potential harms from doing so. It is likely that regular use of heroin will lead to harms, particularly if the substance is consumed illicitly (as it is likely to be), and is injected.

This would in all likelihood impact on an individual's lifestyle, and quality of life, in a negative way, making it harder to hold down work or personal relationships. But long-term addiction isn't as inevitable as it is often perceived.

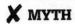 **MYTH**

The drug perpetuates the addiction and circumstance has no effect

It's a theme throughout this book that a huge factor in your experience of taking a drug will be the two S's: set and setting. And so it is with heroin. Researchers have interviewed people who use heroin and found that they experience overdoses more often when consuming the drug in locations where they've not been before, or when circumstances are different. So, the setting is clearly very important here.

It seems that the body somehow 'prepares for' or expects heroin when cues that are associated with using heroin are present in the environment, although how it does this is currently not known. This idea of the importance of setting or circumstance is also vividly shown in research conducted in the USA during and after the Vietnam War, where many soldiers who had become dependent on heroin or opium while serving in Vietnam did not continue to use the drug once they left the war zone and returned to their homes in the USA.*

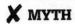 **MYTH**

---

* There's more detail and discussion about this study in the Addiction chapter, should you be interested.

Abstinence is the only cure for heroin addiction

While the only way to ensure that you will not experience any harm from a substance is to not take it, if you want to reduce your risk of harm from heroin without stopping taking it, this is possible. Taking it less regularly, leaving at least a few days between uses or ideally even longer, will reduce the physical dependence on heroin. If you are consuming heroin via injection, then changing to a less immediate method of consumption such as snorting or inhaling will reduce harm, and could help reduce dependence. Similarly, if you do continue injecting, then finding a source of sterilised needles and acid can reduce your risk of harm.

In the UK there are needle and syringe programmes, and there is discussion in Scotland at present to introduce injection rooms, where people can consume the drug as well, rather than having to take sterilised equipment out into non-sterile environments to use ir. Injection rooms have been implemented successfully in many other countries around Europe, including Switzerland, Germany, Spain, Norway and France. Many are opening in Canada in response to the opioid emergency occurring in North America.

If you want to stop taking heroin, then you can get medical help. In the UK, doctors can prescribe heroin substitutes, commonly methadone or buprenorphine (also known as Subutex). Methadone is a synthetic opioid similar to heroin. It is usually administered at selected GP surgeries as a green liquid. Doses are given one at a time, to consume on the premises. As it is similar to heroin, if you continue to use heroin while using methadone, it's easier to overdose.

Buprenorphine is a little different. If you have taken buprenorphine, then this will block the effect of heroin if you take that as well, making it harder (although still possible) to overdose, but also meaning that taking heroin will not be pleasurable anymore. For this reason, people who are prescribed buprenorphine will sometimes stop taking it so that they can resume use of heroin once it has left their system.

It's believed that withdrawal from methadone is less severe than withdrawal from heroin (although the evidence to support this isn't completely conclusive). There is a debate among public health and medical researchers about whether people who have successfully moved from using heroin to using methadone should be maintained on methadone long-term, or whether the goal should be complete withdrawal from everything eventually.

 MYTH

Why is it so hard to stop using heroin?

As we've already mentioned, heroin is dependence forming if used regularly, and withdrawal symptoms are really unpleasant. But often, it's hard for some people to stop using heroin for environmental or external reasons, rather than or as well as the physical dependence. If, after detoxing from heroin, you return to the environment where you've always taken it, the cues that you associate with the drug might make it seem very tempting again.

If your group of friends are using it, and it's easily available, the temptation to use it again will be higher. Heroin is a drug often used by people who have very difficult lives, so unless a person's circumstances change, the urge to use heroin may well remain.

All of these factors can play a role in why it's hard to stop using heroin, and why people relapse even after they are no longer physically dependent on it.

Why do people overdose on heroin?

It's really dangerous to take too much heroin – in severe cases fatal. And for a number of reasons, it's quite easy to do this. Firstly, if you're injecting a drug, there's nothing you can do about altering the level of the dose once you've consumed it – once you've injected it, it's in you. With something like alcohol, if you drink too much, one of the first things that your body does is try to expel this by vomiting. This won't work with heroin, because it's not in the stomach waiting to be absorbed, it's already in the bloodstream. Because of heroin's legal status around the world, it can be even harder to ascertain correctly the dose required, because there's no way of knowing the purity of it, or what it's been mixed with.

Samples of street heroin seized in the UK have been found to be mixed with paracetamol, sugar, and sometimes other sedatives – this can make it extremely unpredictable, as some substances might interact with it and exacerbate the effects of heroin, increasing the risk of overdose or side-effects.* Also, as we've already discussed, the setting in which you consume heroin can impact on the likelihood of overdose, with this being more common in novel settings.

Tolerance to heroin can fall quite quickly if you don't take it for even as short a time as a couple of days. This means if your supply runs out and you can't replenish it straight away, or if for any reason you stop using for a few days, the next time you use it, you'll need to take a smaller dose.

---

* In recent years, heroin laced with fentanyl, a more potent opioid, has been found in circulation. This can greatly increase the risk of overdose.

Does heroin have any medical uses?

While there is an argument to be made that some people use heroin as a means of escape from their circumstances for a few hours, which could be seen as self-medicating, using heroin in this way will be a short-term solution to a long-term problem, and will certainly do an individual more harm than good. While intoxicated on heroin, people may be even less likely to seek help for the problems that led to heroin use in the first place.

However, morphine, a compound very similar to heroin, is extremely useful as pain medication across the world. It is prescribed for acute pain, from heart attacks to cancer, and is likely to be the first choice for prescription unless a person has allergies to it or has previously suffered serious side-effects from it.*

---

* Is it right to prescribe morphine, or other opioids, for non-cancer chronic pain? Some believe over-prescription is in part responsible for the opioid crisis that countries like the USA and Canada are experiencing. This is covered in more detail in the Prescription Opioids chapter.

Focus on: Drugs and Mental Health

There is a strong link between drug use and mental health problems. This is true of a lot of substances, including alcohol, cigarettes and cannabis, and it's true of a number of different mental health problems, including depression, anxiety and even more serious conditions such as psychosis or schizophrenia.

We know this because we see substance use at higher levels in people with poor mental health. We also see rates of poor mental health at higher levels among people who use substances, and people who are heavier users of substances, than people who don't use them.

The difficult thing is untangling what this association means. It could be one of a few different things, or potentially some combination of all of them.

Drug use causes poor mental health?

The first interpretation is that taking a substance causes an increase in risk for poor mental health. There's some evidence that points in this direction. We know that psychoactive substances impact on some of the brain pathways and neurotransmitters that we think are also implicated in poor mental health, which could be an explanation. Also, substance use has often started before poor mental health symptoms are reported, which would suggest causality is going in that direction.

People with poor mental health seek out drugs?

Another explanation for an association between drugs and mental health could be that people with poor mental health are more likely to use drugs because of their poor mental health. This explanation also makes a lot of sense. When people are asked about their motivation to use substances, a lot report doing so 'to cope' – we see this with alcohol, opioids, and other substances, too. If a drug can numb painful feelings, help a person to get to sleep, or even just provide a break from unpleasant thoughts, it's easy to see why people might turn to it. Particularly in a society where we don't have perfect treatments or support for people experiencing difficulties with their mental health, and where many people go untreated.

Earlier life factors influence both, and the association is just coincidence?

There's a third possibility as to why we see a link between drugs and mental health. It could be that factors, be they genetic or environmental, might influence both things, and the link we see between the two is simply an artefact of something else going on. There's also some evidence to back this idea up. Early-life or childhood trauma is a strong predictor of both a likelihood to use psychoactive substances, and a likelihood to experience poor mental health. And there might be loads of other factors that could influence this, too.

Untangling it all

Working out which of these is the true reason for the association between drugs and mental health is really hard. And I speak from personal experience here: my research is specifically trying to unpick this question, and I've been doing it for over a decade now – and I don't have any definitive answers yet. My hunch, though, which is evidence-based as much as it can be, is that in all likelihood it's a combination of all of these possible explanations.

People who are predisposed biologically or environmentally to use a substance are also those who are at a higher risk of poor mental health. They might start using a substance initially to deal with difficult symptoms, but unfortunately the substance might be effective in the short-term, but make matters worse in the long term.

What's also important to note is that these associations get stronger when we focus particularly on the people who are dependent on a substance, or have problematic patterns of use. This would also fit with this working hypothesis – we know that when a person starts to rely on a substance, this can be an indicator of increasing risk of harm, in terms of dependence or addiction, but also in terms of other difficult factors in their life that maybe are not being addressed.

CHAPTER 12

Ketamine

What is it? Yes, it really is a horse tranquiliser, but it's also got a lot of other uses. A synthetic substance developed as an anaesthetic in the 1960s, on the WHO's list of essential medicines.

Type of drug: Depressant – a dissociative anaesthetic.

Popularity: Used in veterinary and human medicine, but also recreationally.

How consumed: Snorted, or occasionally smoked or injected (under the skin).

Timescale: Quick onset, intoxication can last for a couple of hours.

Some effects: Stimulating at low dose, mild psychedelic effects at moderate dose, impact on cognitive abilities, confusion, amnesia, severe impact on movement at high doses.

KETAMINE HYDROCHLORIDE IS a synthetic dissociative anaesthetic. Those aren't necessarily words you hear together that often, so let's unpick this a bit. Synthetic means created by people, rather than being extracted from something naturally occurring (usually a plant). Anaesthetic is probably a word you're familiar with – these are drugs that numb parts of the body, or cause a person to fall asleep, enabling medical procedures that would otherwise cause pain or discomfort to be conducted.

But how is it dissociative? Dissociation is a feeling of being disconnected from your thoughts or feelings, or your sense of identity. Dissociative anaesthetics do not necessarily lead a person to lose consciousness, but they induce an inability to move or feel. Ketamine is on the World Health Organisation's list of essential medicine, and it's the most widely used anaesthetic in veterinary medicine across the world – colloquially it has been known as 'the horse tranquiliser', but it's used with a variety of small and medium-sized mammals.

But we are not here to talk about horses (though we will explore veterinary use of K a little more later in the chapter, if you're interested). Recreationally, ketamine is usually consumed by snorting the substance as a white crystalline powder, at lower doses than when it's used as an anaesthetic. However, it can also be injected, usually under the skin rather than into the bloodstream, or smoked. It is sometimes used in a club setting, but also for its psychedelic effects.

What are the short-term effects?

When ketamine is snorted, it gets into the bloodstream quickly, and because of this the intoxication effects occur soon after it's taken. Although it's an anaesthetic, it has differing effects depending on the amount a person consumes, and at low doses it raises the heart rate, and can – counterintuitively for an anaesthetic – make an individual feel more energised. Even in small amounts, ketamine can impact on a person's ability to speak properly, and to perform some basic cognitive processes, such as spatial awareness and perception.

A number of people I spoke to described ketamine intoxication as making things go 'a bit slanty'. One person described feeling like 'the floor had become made of sponge cake, and it was really difficult to walk through the cake'.

It's also associated with cognitive impairment during intoxication, including to speech and executive function – the brain functions involved in planning and executing complex tasks. Ketamine can cause amnesia, and other memory problems.

Ketamine intoxication can induce mild psychedelic effects, such as perceptual changes and psychotic-like experiences, which are appealing to some users, but can also be distressing. Lucy described 'mini fireworks on things, like when you look into a kaleidoscope you get shimmery shapes. Or when you see car headlights in a rear-view mirror in the rain.' 'Diffraction halos' is the term she created to describe them.

At slightly higher doses, users can experience a dissociative state, where their mind feels separated from their body. This can also manifest as a feeling of depersonalisation – a sensation where a person's thoughts and feelings feel like they don't belong to themselves, or they belong to someone else. Hence the 'dissociation' in dissociative anaesthetic.

At higher doses still, the anaesthetic quality of ketamine becomes more pronounced. People who have consumed these quantities may find it difficult to move, and may feel that their limbs are heavy. They may also find their ability to feel pain is reduced, and they might feel numb.

At this level of intoxication an individual can experience more vivid hallucinations. Some people describe what is known in some circles as 'the K-hole', where ability to move or speak is greatly impaired, and the intoxication experience is directed inwards, as a spiritual or gnostic experience. People report intoxication experiences where they feel a heightened connection to the world, or out-of-body or near-death experiences that can be extremely rich in detail.

The anaesthetic property of ketamine is a particular risk for people who take ketamine recreationally: people consuming higher doses are vulnerable to assault from others while they are in this state, or they might put themselves in danger by not being aware of their surroundings – being unaware they are outside and it is cold can lead to hypothermia, or being unaware of surroundings could lead to walking into traffic.

When I used to live in Bristol, there was an apocryphal tale about a group of people who had taken ketamine running around the city centre with a frying pan, asking passers-by to whack them over the head with it, cartoon-style. I think this is extremely unlikely to be true, but if it was, they certainly might not feel the pain that evening (although, in the morning . . .). But I don't mean to make light of this, I've also heard from other individuals who have been assaulted or raped and unable to resist, due to their inability to move or their lack of full consciousness, while on ketamine.

If you are considering taking high doses of ketamine to ex-perience 'the K-hole', it's extremely important to ensure you are in a safe place, and that there is someone else present to look after you, before you do so.

Ketamine can become more dangerous still when mixed with other substances. Because of its anaesthetic qualities, it's dangerous to use ketamine alongside depressants such as alcohol or opiates, as this can substantially increase the risk of passing out, stopping breathing or choking on vomit. It's also important to avoid mixing ketamine and most allergy medication (antihistamines), as they can increase dizziness, drowsiness, confusion and inability to concentrate.

Despite these risks, ketamine is a drug that people often report using in combination with other drugs. In particular, people I spoke to told me they used ketamine to extend a psychedelic trip, or in combination with cocaine, although this is ill-advised as taking ketamine alongside stimulants can put extra pressure on the heart, and also increase the risk of anxiety brought on by heightened arousal, and can lead to symptoms such as palpitations.

What are the longer-term effects?

There are a growing number of anecdotal reports and case studies showing that heavy ketamine use is associated with bladder and urinary tract problems, in particular a type of ulcerative cystitis called ketamine-induced ulcerative cystitis. This is an extremely unpleasant disorder, with symptoms including bladder pain, blood in urine, a constant need to urinate but often finding it difficult to go, pain such as burning when urinating, and needing to urinate throughout the night.

Although the mechanism by which ketamine might cause these problems isn't well known, there is some evidence from case studies of heavy recreational ketamine users that daily use for prolonged periods of time might lead to the thickening of the bladder wall. Other evidence suggests that ketamine has a direct effect on the lining of the bladder. Heavy users sometimes report cloudy or bloody urine, pain when going to the toilet, and urge incontinence. Urinary problems are extremely rare in individuals who have been prescribed ketamine for medical reasons, but a growing problem in heavy recreational users.

It is not only the bladder at risk from heavy ketamine use. There are also a number of reports of kidney dysfunction, and what are referred to as 'K-cramps' – extreme abdominal pain that some have hypothesised may be linked to liver damage (although this is unclear at the moment). It becomes a vicious cycle as people then report using ketamine to numb the pain of these cramps.

There is some evidence that prolonged heavy ketamine use is associated with memory problems. Interestingly, a small study of eighteen ketamine users and ten polydrug-using controls also found some evidence that semantic memory impairments seen in ketamine users may reverse if a person dramatically cuts down their use. The study tested individuals at baseline and then three to four years later on the same battery of tests. Over that time period, the average reduction of ketamine use in the study was 88 per cent.

However, the same study found little evidence that impairments to episodic memory and attention improved, and the same was true of reports of lingering perceptual distortions and sub-clinical, schizophrenia-esque thoughts.

As with many of these studies, it is difficult to know with certainty whether or not there were already pre-existing differences between those who use ketamine, and those who choose not to, but the use of a control group who also use other substances is an attempt to minimise this problem, as they are likely to be more similar to people who use ketamine than are people who don't use any substances.

Ketamine appears to be dependence forming to some heavy users, although this is hard to ascertain for certain as large-scale investigations have not been conducted. However, ketamine has a number of properties such as fast onset and short-lasting effect that are linked to risk of habit-forming.

It is also the case that tolerance to the drug can build up, meaning higher doses are required for a regular or even infrequent user to get the same effect, which can then go on to increase the risk of bladder damage, and perpetuate the vicious cycle of using ketamine to numb the pain that overuse of the drug itself is causing. Compulsive behaviour is also reported by some individuals that use ketamine – who have stated that they will keep taking it until their supply runs out.

There are risks specific to injecting ketamine – if injecting under the muscle, this can lead to irritation and damage to the skin at the site of injection.

Myths and misconceptions

Ketamine is a horse tranquiliser

This is pretty much true – it's an extremely useful anaesthetic in veterinary medicine, for small and large animals, though it's not specifically a horse tranquiliser. The World Health Organisation reports that ketamine is the most widely used veterinary anaesthetic across the globe. It's particularly useful in locations where people are trying to manage populations of feral animals. Because ketamine can be administered via injection under the muscle, it can be done so via a dart gun from a distance, or a needle through the bars of a cage, putting people at less risk of transmitted diseases such as rabies.

Even in the UK, ketamine can be used to anaesthetise an angry cat through the bars of a cage, rather than risk handling the animal and getting scratched or bitten. However, it's important here to think about the difference between a tranquiliser and an anaesthetic.

Tranquilisers, or sedatives, are useful to relax and becalm an animal, but don't necessarily knock an animal out or act to prevent it feeling pain, the way an anaesthetic does.

Because of ketamine's safety profile, it makes a good animal anaesthetic – and this is of particular importance to horses, as their size and fragility mean there are extra complications when knocking out a horse.

You need to lie it down carefully, and if the horse is laid down for a long time, there is a risk that its body muscle can constrict its lungs. Horses' hearts also beat slowly in normal circumstances, so anaesthetics that further slow the heart rate are extremely dangerous. Rather than bringing a horse into a specialised surgery with equipment to allow anaesthesia via gas, ketamine can be used to anaesthetise a horse in the field (sometimes literally, or else at a clinic without full gas anaesthesia equipment).

Ketamine's beneficial use here is probably why it became known as a horse tranquiliser. Although apparently it is also extremely useful in camel surgery. And it's also useful in situations where it is challenging to weigh an animal to estimate the dose required for anaesthesia. Because it doesn't depress breathing or impact on heart rate, if the dose is slightly overestimated this will not put the animal in undue danger – ketamine has what's known as a 'large window of efficacy', meaning there is a lot of headroom in dosing before risking overdose.

However, whether an individual veterinary surgery will use ketamine or not is quite variable – veterinary medicine is less controlled than human medicine, meaning protocols vary across sites.

Dr Danny Chambers is a vet who has worked in a number of locations in north and south-west England. He told me that in some practices, ketamine would be used very regularly, and in others hardly at all, although he doesn't recall working anywhere without ketamine onsite.

He also told me about the procedures and protocols that need to be followed in order to use ketamine, due to its use as a recreational drug. If he needs to take ketamine out to treat a horse (for example), he needs to sign it out, and keep it in a locked case in his vehicle. If he uses any to treat an animal, this needs to be detailed when he signs it back in. When working out of hours, at the start and end of a shift, the ketamine on site must be weighed, and any use must be recorded, to prevent any going missing. It is kept in a 'dangerous medicines' locked cabinet.

There are more legal regulations around the storage of drugs with abuse potential, such as ketamine and morphine, than there are around the drugs that vets use for euthanasia. (Although often the drugs are treated the same by individual practices, there is no legal obligation for them to do so.)

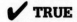 **TRUE**

Does ketamine have any medical uses?

Ketamine was first synthesised in the early 1960s for human medical use. At the time, PCP was being used as an anaesthetic, but had a pretty bad adverse event profile, so researchers were looking for a drug that was similar but with less unpleasant side-effects. Ketamine was synthesised in the USA and was initially tested in the prison population there, where it was found to be more appropriate for use in humans than PCP. It was given approval by the FDA (the USA's Food and Drug Administration) in 1970, and one of its first wide usages was to US soldiers during the Vietnam War.

Ketamine is extremely useful as an anaesthetic in locations where ventilation equipment isn't available. Although its slight psychedelic effects don't make it an ideal anaesthetic in general, it doesn't impact on breathing rates as much as other anaesthetics do, so it is extremely useful in the field, or in locations where it's harder to access such equipment. Because it doesn't lower blood pressure, it's also useful as a pain medication (analgesic) in emergency trauma situations.

Finally, because it can be injected rather than needing to be administered as a gas, it's more portable than many other anaesthetics, meaning it's often used by emergency services in order to stabilise a patient while they are brought to hospital.

Although it's not fully understood why, it seems that children aren't likely to experience the hallucinations and delusions associated with ketamine that adults do, so it used to be popular in paediatric medicine as well. However, although ketamine was deemed less problematic than PCP in terms of side-effects, it was still found to induce hallucinations, vivid dreams, and dysphoria – a feeling of unhappiness or unwellness – and so other anaesthetics are now preferred. That said, ketamine is still to this day an extremely widely used anaesthetic worldwide.

The World Health Organisation lists it as an essential medicine, and it's prescribed in low doses for the treatment of pain, particularly nerve pain (sometimes called neuropathic pain). It's used in palliative care, and in treatment for chronic cancer pain – particularly for individuals who are no longer responding to conventional opioid pain treatment.

Ketamine also has a further use in medical research. The impact that it can have on a person's state of mind has been likened to that seen in patients with schizophrenia. This includes not only the positive symptoms of schizophrenia, such as hallucinations and delusions, but also what are known as the negative symptoms – an inability to feel pleasure, or withdrawal – and the cognitive impairments (ketamine has been shown to lead to amnesia after consumption, and there's some evidence that it impacts spatial awareness).

As such, researchers are looking to ketamine to try and understand what might cause schizophrenia. As yet, if anything it has thrown up more questions than it's answered, but as we understand more about how ketamine impacts on the brain, this could also help us to understand what brain changes might lead to serious and impairing conditions like schizophrenia.

What don't we know?

There's some suggestion that ketamine could be effective for treatment-resistant depression, a notoriously difficult condition to treat (hence the name). A pilot study conducted in Oxford in 2014 gave twenty-eight patients with severe treatment-resistant depression, or bipolar disorder, low doses of intravenous (IV) ketamine infusion of varying concentrations, over a period of three weeks. The results were mixed, with eight individuals responding well to the treatment for between twenty-five days and twenty-four weeks. However, eight other people in the study didn't complete the treatment, either because they suffered adverse reactions to the infusion, or because they were not experiencing any benefit and were becoming more anxious.

In 2017, at the appositely named Black Dog Institute in Sydney, Australia, a randomised controlled trial of IV ketamine found it to be well-tolerated and potentially effective in a group of elderly patients with treatment-resistant depression, although again it was a small-scale investigatory study, so cannot tell us too much about its effectiveness.

More recently, Yale School of Medicine ran a study in collaboration with a pharmaceutical company to investigate the impact of a ketamine nasal spray on extremely severe depression – the study recruited sixty-eight people deemed at imminent risk of suicide. The individuals were brought into hospital and given conventional anti-depressants. As well as this, half were given a nasal spray containing esketamine – a ketamine derivative – and half were given a placebo nasal spray.

The study found that depression symptoms were quickly reduced in the patients given esketamine compared to placebo, but any difference between groups had disappeared within a month. The authors suggest that ketamine could be very useful in reducing acute severe depression – current pharmacological depression treatments such as SSRIs are notorious for the lag between beginning treatment and an impact on depression being felt, which can take a few weeks. If ketamine is effective in giving some respite to people suffering, while other treatments can kick in, it could be really helpful and save lives.

However, not all researchers are equally optimistic. Another study attempted to investigate the same question using nasal spray, but was forced to end prematurely as patients with treatment-resistant depression recruited into the study were unable to self-administer the doses required before losing coordination abilities, and some showed poor tolerability to ketamine. The group also found a huge variation in the levels of ketamine and its metabolites in the blood of individuals who had been administered the same dose. Having said that, esketamine nasal spray is now licensed in the USA for prescription for treatment-resistant depression. At the moment it's marketed under the brand names Ketanest and Spravato, among others.

Ketamine is also currently being investigated as a treatment for alcohol addiction, by a team based in Exeter in the southwest of England, led by Professor Celia Morgan. The concept that ketamine could be used in this way is not a new one. Experiments were initially conducted in the 1980s in Russia, where individuals with severe alcohol dependence were given a dose of ketamine once a week for three weeks, alongside psychological therapy. These individuals were compared to a group who received only treatment as usual. After a year, 66 per cent of the individuals given ketamine were still alcohol abstinent, while only 24 per cent of the other group were.

This study design wasn't ideal – control participants were just given treatment as normal, meaning it was clear to both the participants and the experimenters who was in which group. The new study, which is ongoing at the time I'm writing this, is recruiting individuals with problematic alcohol use who have made the decision to give up alcohol completely. They will be administering a placebo to the control group, and neither researchers nor participants will know which group they are in – known as a 'double blind' study.

But why might ketamine improve depression, and improve the chances of people trying to abstain from alcohol being able to do so? Animal studies in rats have suggested that perhaps ketamine might stimulate brain growth. Rats given ketamine were found to show increased levels of a protein called BDNF – brain-derived neurotrophic factor. This protein is implicated in the growth of neurons, or brain cells. Whether this is the case for humans has yet to be established. However, some researchers believe that it is the intoxication effect itself that might be the mechanism by which ketamine has these potential benefits.

This theory became particularly prominent after other compounds that were very similar to ketamine, but without a psychoactive element, were successfully trialled in animals, but did not produce the desired results in human trials. Perhaps there's something about the 'mystical' intoxication effects that is important. This is also something that's been proposed as to why psychedelics such as magic mushrooms and LSD might be useful as treatments for depression.

We're a long way from knowing whether this is the case, but it's one possible explanation for potentially yet another effect of this often-misunderstood substance.

CHAPTER 13

Khat

CATHINE OH

CATHINONE O

What is it? Leaf that grows in the Horn of Africa and the Arabian Peninsula.

Type of drug: Cathinone is a stimulant.

Popularity: Popular among Yemeni and Somali populations, particularly men.

How consumed: Fresh leaves are chewed, dried leaves can be made into tea.

Timescale: Slow onset, long-lasting as it can be chewed continuously.

Some effects: Similar to a strong coffee – positive mood, sociability, jittery, lower appetite, insomnia.

KHAT (CATHA EDULIS) is a plant, known by many names around the world, which grows in the Horn of Africa and the Arabian Peninsula. The leaves are bitter tasting, and when chewed release cathinone and its metabolite cathine, two stimulants. Khat's legality varies across the world – it is not scheduled under the UN's Single

Convention on Narcotic Drugs, despite being classified by the World Health Organisation as a drug of abuse in 1980.

Some countries such as the UK, much of the rest of Europe, a number of Middle Eastern countries and China, have chosen to make khat a controlled substance. In other places such as Yemen, Ethiopia, Somalia and a number of other East African countries, khat is legal. It is used in some cultures as part of a religious-type ceremony. The leader will use khat to induce a fuller spiritual connection.

Khat use is often a communal activity – and until the ban in 2014, it was popular among East African communities living in the UK. In those communities it is predominantly consumed by men, who will meet up to consume khat and socialise. In some parts of the UK there were 'khat cafés', particularly popular with Somali communities, while Yemeni communities in the UK would often use khat in private homes and social locations.

Khat is usually fresh when it is chewed, because the cathinone in the leaves quickly turns into the less potent cathine if the leaves are left to sit. It is possible to make tea from dried khat, but it will be much less potent than fresh leaves.

What are the short-term effects?

To consume khat, fresh leaves are balled up into a wad, which will be chewed by an individual for at least an hour. Over the course of a session (for want of a better word) on khat, usually a couple of wads will be chewed. Cathinone, and its metabolite cathine, are mild stimulants, and intoxication on khat is broadly similar in magnitude to that you'd experience from a strong coffee, or a low dose of a stimulant like amphetamine. People who use khat report feeling increased wellbeing, including chattiness and a positive mood. It's these intoxication effects that make it popular in social settings.

Like other stimulants, chewing khat can increase alertness, but can also make a person feel more jittery. It will increase heart rate and blood pressure, while it will suppress appetite, and it may impact on ability to sleep, similar to caffeine. Because it is chewed, khat intoxication has a slow onset – similar to chewing coca leaf. It is very hard to overdose on khat when consuming it in this way, as it's almost impossible to chew the amount of leaves required for a toxic dose. There's weak evidence that khat intoxication could slightly increase the risk of heart attack – probably due to it being a mild stimulant and increasing heart rate and blood pressure. However, the evidence base is very limited, and any increased risk is likely to be small.

What are the longer-term effects?

As with many substances discussed in this book, far less is known definitively about the longer-term impact of using khat. Although its use is legal in many countries around the world, khat is still nowhere near as widely used as, say, alcohol is in Europe and the USA. Khat is often consumed in social settings where people might also be smoking tobacco, and consuming sugary, fizzy drinks. This can make it harder to tease out whether any health problems seen in people who regularly use khat are due to the khat itself, or to other aspects of their behaviour or environment.

The populations who regularly use khat may also be individuals who find it hard to access health services, so this could also impact on their general health. For example, heavy khat use has been linked to respiratory problems, but only when users also smoke or spend time in smoky environments. As is the case with many other substances, people who use khat rarely do so without the use of any other substances, and the effects of them might interact.

People who regularly use khat report a mild comedown after

having used it, including mood swings, and feeling grumpy and irritable. However, it's unclear whether regular khat use leads to tolerance.

When people stop using khat after having used for a long time, they can report lethargy, mild depression, slight trembling and some may experience recurring bad dreams. At the moment there's little evidence to suggest that khat might be dependence forming – we can't conclude either way at present. Case studies have identified individuals who would be categorised as dependent on the substance, but whether this would hold at a population level is harder to say.

It's important to highlight here again that individuals who use khat might be less likely to seek medical help if experiencing dependence, which could then mean that their problems are not recorded when prevalence information is collected, which could in turn make it seem like khat is less addictive than it actually is. In the UK, mental health services are less accessible for members of Black, Asian and minority ethnic (BAME) communities than for their white counterparts, and khat is almost exclusively used by minority ethnic individuals.

There's some evidence from animal studies, and some case reports in humans, of khat use being linked to liver problems. However, any association is far from clear. There have been cases where individuals have developed liver problems severe enough to require liver transplants, although only in small numbers. Unusually, although linked to khat use, these problems don't seem to be predicted by heaviness of use or other patterns that might be expected to predict physical health problems. As yet, it's not clear why some individuals seem particularly susceptible to liver damage from khat, or whether there are other factors at play that so far haven't been identified.

Khat use has been linked to oral cancers and oral health more generally, much like chewing tobacco. These suggestive findings are based on small studies, and while it seems there may be changes in the mucous membrane that lines the mouth of regular khat chewers, whether these changes increase the risk of oral cancers has not been proven.

Interestingly, in the UK, dental problems are seen at higher rates in people who use khat, including cavities. However dental problems of this kind are not seen in populations in the Yemen who use khat, which has led some to conclude that it is due to the use of sugary, fizzy drinks to counteract the bitter taste of the leaves – a practice popular in the UK but not in Yemen. Comparing the relationship between khat and an outcome like tooth decay in two populations where other behaviours are different can be useful when trying to work out whether the cause might be the substance itself, or something else (in this case, sugary drinks).

There have also been case reports of people experiencing acute psychotic episodes after using khat. This is something that is seen with a number of other psychostimulants, such as amphetamine, so perhaps this is not surprising. Clinicians have also reported that treatment of mental ill health can be complicated if an individual is also using khat, although these are just anecdotal reports. Analysis is complicated in the UK as most people who chew khat are from an immigrant population with high levels of underlying trauma. These factors in themselves predispose people to higher rates of mental illness – not only that, but the types of mental illnesses that are harder to treat effectively.

As yet there is no robust evidence to determine whether khat has a causal relationship on its own for mental illness. In populations with high levels of khat-chewing in society, such as Yemen, there is not a higher rate of mental illness than other similar non-khat using populations. This suggests that at a broad population level, there is no association with khat use and mental illness.

Myths and misconceptions

Khat's not a drug – it's more like coffee, or alcohol

Likening khat to coffee is not far off in terms of its intoxication effect. But as we know, caffeine and alcohol are drugs! And not considering a substance as a drug can be problematic if a person does get ill. For example, if a person presents to their doctor with liver problems and is asked 'Do you use drugs?' they might answer 'No', meaning the doctor will not consider the impact of khat on their liver, and the problem might go undiagnosed while their condition deteriorates.

✗ MYTH

Khat is the 'natural' version of synthetic cathinones like mephedrone or MDPV

This is somewhat of a complicated one. Mephedrone and other related drugs are often called 'synthetic cathinones', but more technically they are methcathinones. All these drugs are stimulants, so their effects are certainly similar. But chewing khat means cathinone will be released slowly, and at a low concentration. Not only that, but because of the bulk of plant material chewed, it is very difficult to get quickly a high dose of cathinone or cathine from khat.

This is markedly different from consuming mephedrone or other synthetic cathinones as a powder, either swallowed or snorted, where doses are likely to be much higher and to reach the brain faster, meaning the intoxication experience will be different, but the risk of taking too much is also higher.

? PARTLY TRUE

Does khat have any medical uses?

Khat is not used in Western medicine, and there doesn't seem to be any evidence that it ever has been. However, in north-east Africa it is used to treat a number of conditions, including depression and gastric ulcer. Its stimulant effects mean it is used to treat tiredness. It is also offered to individuals who are hungry but cannot access all the food they need, as it can suppress appetite. For this reason, it is also used to treat obesity.

Focus on: Drugs and the Brain

Throughout this book there are lots of references to neurotransmitters, synapses, receptors, and other brain-related terms. It is quite well understood that psychoactive drugs have an effect on the brain – but how?

Neuroscience 101

Ignoring drugs for a moment, how do our brains work? To be slightly over-simplistic, they are kind of like very complex electrical circuits, or networks might be a better analogy. We each have billions of brain cells (neurons – current estimates put the number at around 100 billion), and each is connected to billions of other neurons (our brains are thought to have around 100 trillion connections). Electrical impulses occur when a neuron gets enough of a signal from the neurons around it, and then it'll pass that signal on to the other neurons surrounding it. The signal is passed across the synapse – the gap between neurons – by chemicals called neurotransmitters. Our brains are passing signals around like this all the time, even while we are asleep, controlling everything from our breathing to our dreaming.

There are a number of different types of neurotransmitter that our brains use for different types of signal, and they're all molecules of different shapes. These neurotransmitters fit into differently shaped receptors on the surface of the next neuron in the chain – the analogy used is often like a key in a lock – and the next neuron will fire, passing the message along.

Different neurotransmitters seem to be involved in different brain functions, and different neuronal pathways around the brain. Dopamine is one often mentioned when talking about drugs – it's thought to be involved in reward and reinforcement of behaviours, motivation, and motor control. Serotonin is also linked to drug use. This neurotransmitter is linked to many high-level brain functions such as mood and memory, as well as other important behaviours like sleep and appetite. Some neurotransmitters do the opposite and inhibit the firing of the next neuron – GABA is an example of this kind of neurotransmitter. Other neurotransmitters you might have heard of include noradrenaline, histamine and acetylcholine.

What happens when psychoactive substances are added into the mix?

Psychoactive substances tend to affect the brain in one of three ways, all of which involve neurotransmitters. Some drugs have a very similar molecular shape to certain natural (endogenous) neurotransmitters already present in our bodies or brains. DMT, for example, is a similarly shaped molecule to serotonin. Cannabinoids found in cannabis are a similar shape to the endocannabinoids we make. Opioids are similar to endorphins.

In these cases, molecules of the drug can fit on to the receptors for these neurotransmitters, but here's where the key-in-the lock analogy slightly falls down. Because these molecules aren't exactly the same shape as our own neurotransmitters, the effects that they have on the receptors and neurons they bind to is slightly different. They don't just have the same effect as our own neurotransmitters, and so we experience a psychoactive effect.

Other drugs change the levels of our existing neurotransmitters. Cocaine, amphetamine and MDMA are examples of these types of drug. They can have this effect in a couple of ways. They might lead to more neurotransmitter than usual being released into the synaptic cleft (the gap between two neurons). Or they might block the action of the mechanism that collects up and recycles the neurotransmitters that don't bind to receptors. Either way, the upshot is that the space between neurons ends up with more neurotransmitter present, which can lead to overstimulation or disruption of the usual communication pathways between neurons, and a psychoactive effect.

CHAPTER 14
Kratom

MITRAGYNINE

HYDROXYMITRAGYNINE

What is it? Leaves of a tree that grows in Southeast
Asia.

Type of drug: Depressant (sedative), though can have
stimulant-like effects at low dose.

Popularity: Historically used in Southeast Asia, but recently
growing in popularity in the USA.

How consumed: Fresh leaves are chewed, or powder is made
into a tea.

Timescale: Onset around 30 minutes, can last 4 to 6 hours.

Some effects: Stimulating at low dose, euphoria and relaxation.
Sedation and pain relief at higher doses, dizziness and
nausea, constipation or stomach upset.

I MUST ADMIT that I hadn't heard of kratom before I started
making the *Say Why to Drugs* podcast. But it's probably the
substance I received the most messages about – asking for an
episode, or for more information. Kratom is the colloquial name

for the leaves of the tropical evergreen tree *Mitragyna speciosa*. The tree, in the coffee family, grows in Southeast Asia.

Across the region, kratom has been used as a herbal remedy for hundreds of years, for all sorts of ailments from diarrhoea to aches and pains, from coughs to being used as a wound poultice. The bitter leaves are usually mixed with salt (to prevent constipation) and chewed, although dried leaves can also be steeped in hot water to make a tea, often sweetened or mixed with sweeter beverages such as fizzy drinks to improve their bitter taste.

In recent years, kratom use has grown in popularity, particularly in the USA. It's hard to get a good estimate as to how many people in the USA are using kratom, but a pro-kratom lobby group have estimated that around 5 million people are regular users in the country. It is particularly popular, according to the group, among people who are experiencing symptoms of anxiety or pain, and to a lesser extent among people trying to cut down their use of opioids. They found it is most commonly being used by white, middle-aged, employed men.

Chewing kratom leaves is also popular in Southeast Asia among people working in manual-labour occupations, similarly to how khat and coca leaves (cocaine) are used in other regions, to provide energy and to improve mood. In the USA, kratom is most often available as a powdered extract, which can be dissolved into a drink, or consumed along with food.

What is it?

Kratom researchers broadly agree that there are two psychoactive compounds in kratom leaves – mitragynine and 7-hydroxymitragynine. Research into these compounds is in its infancy, although growing. Both mitragynine and 7-hydroxymitragynine seem to have pain-relieving properties. 7-hydroxymitragynine might be the compound that leads to reinforcement, and potentially a risk of dependence – at present there is no evidence that mitragynine is dependence forming. However, there are many other alkaloids present in the leaves, which might also impact on the intoxication experience.

People who use kratom recreationally report that they do so because they like the feelings of alertness and confidence it gives, with some likening the intoxication experience to that of alcohol.

What are the short-term effects?

If chewing or drinking kratom, intoxication onset will occur around fifteen to thirty minutes after consumption, and effects can last for four to six hours. At low doses, kratom appears to act like a stimulant, and people report feeling energised and talkative. People might also experience euphoria and relaxation. At higher doses, the effects of kratom appear to be more sedative and analgesic (pain relieving). People may feel nauseous or dizzy, comparing the sensation to that of an alcohol hangover. High doses can lead to vomiting. People have reported having vivid dreams after taking kratom. Kratom intoxication can cause constipation and stomach irritability.

There's very little research into kratom – most of the academic papers published that mention the substance are individual case studies detailing one particular person's experience, which makes it extremely difficult to make generalisations. However, there is some suggestion that heavy regular use of kratom can induce mild depressive symptoms. Similarly, there's some evidence, although not a lot, that regular use can lead to dependence.

Surveys of regular kratom users conducted in both the USA and in Southeast Asia found that these individuals report no impairment of social functioning or cognitive abilities due to their use. Reasons for using were also quite varied – in the USA, people often reported using kratom because they were suffering from mood disorders such as depression and anxiety, although using kratom to deal with withdrawal symptoms from prescription or other, illicit drugs was also reported in this population, as well as for use in pain management.

What are the longer-term effects?

If a person stops using kratom after having previously consumed it regularly, they can report experiencing withdrawal symptoms. These can include things like sweating, nausea, restlessness and difficulty sleeping. Some people report frequent yawning, and having a runny nose. Usually these symptoms will cease by around seven days, although again there's very little research to back up these anecdotal experiences.

A couple of surveys, conducted in Malaysia, where kratom use has occurred for many decades, found that regular users report withdrawal symptoms lasting between one and four days. While these can be unpleasant, they are rated by individuals, their family and healthcare providers as being less severe than opioid withdrawal.

Some reports have suggested that jaundice is a risk from regular use of kratom. Evidence has come from two cases reported in the academic literature. In one of these cases, the individual had also consumed a number of other substances, while in the other the person reported using no other substances, including alcohol. However, the doses the person reported using were, according to the case study, approximately twice the 'usual dosage' reported by others. It's impossible to draw conclusions on the risk of jaundice from just two case studies like this, but they do suggest that it is possible that kratom might pose a risk of liver damage, particularly at extremely high doses.

Similarly, there are case reports of psychosis after use of kratom. Again, without larger-scale studies it's impossible to tell whether kratom was the cause, or whether there were other underlying predictors of psychosis that the individuals had, or even whether the kratom these individuals used was adulterated with other substances.

When kratom is bought as a dried leaf, it may have been sprayed or coated with another substance. Indeed, there have been a number of cases reported where substances believed to be kratom have been found to be mixed with O-desmethyltramadol (a metabolite of the opioid tramadol). And it's this mix of kratom and O-desmethyltramadol – sold as a substance called 'Krypton' – that was implicated in nine deaths that occurred in Sweden, rather than kratom itself. In the USA as of 2016 there have been thirty deaths where kratom was mentioned as having been consumed by the individual, but in all of these cases, other substances had also been consumed.

Experimental studies have found that giving extremely large concentrations of kratom to mice does lead to death, but at quantities around ten times higher than the level of dose that would induce intoxication. There are also some uncertainties about the relevance of these findings to humans, as there is growing evidence that mice metabolise mitragynine differently from larger animals including dogs, monkeys . . . and humans. This phenomenon, called allometric scaling, occurs for some substances, and may mean kratom studies in mice might be limited in how much they can tell us about effects in humans.

Myths and misconceptions

Kratom is an opioid

While there's some suggestion that kratom has its effect in the brain via various types of opioid receptors, that doesn't necessarily mean it's an opioid – ketamine, for example, has an influence on opioid receptors, but wouldn't be called an opioid. The USA's

Food and Drug Administration (FDA) Commissioner has recently stated that he believes that kratom is an opioid, with the potential for dependence, abuse and serious health consequences including death. However, kratom researchers publishing in the journal *Addiction* disagree. They wrote a letter to the editor stating that the evidence available on kratom to date does not support this statement by the FDA Commissioner, although they agree that further research is needed to understand the substance better.

? PROBABLY MYTH

Does kratom have any medical uses?

As yet, there is no good-quality evidence that kratom has any medical benefits. Having said that, as well as the ways in which kratom is used in Southeast Asia as a herbal medicine, many people across the world report using kratom to self-medicate their attempts to withdraw from opiates, such as heroin or prescription opioids. Researchers, particularly in the USA, have been suggesting in recent years that kratom could represent a method of harm reduction in the so-called opioid crisis currently occurring in the USA, given that kratom does not impact on the ability to breathe in the same way that opioids do.

However, as detailed above, there are risks from kratom due to the potential for it to be cut with adulterants, and as yet there is little research into the impact of long-term use other than self-report questionnaires. Also, it is likely that kratom has its own withdrawal symptoms, and even if these are not as extreme as those from opioids, this should not be ignored.

As well as people reporting using kratom to deal with opioid withdrawal, some individuals claim that it helps them manage symptoms of post-traumatic stress disorder. As yet, there is no research into this, and therefore no evidence at all to support kratom as being useful for this. Many people who use kratom also report that it has pain-relieving properties, and given its potential mechanism of effect is on opioid receptors in the brain, the same as a number of other substances that relieve pain (most notably opioids themselves), this is plausible.

So far, the only research to back this up comes from surveys where poly-substance users were asked about their opioid and kratom use. However, there was substantial pushback from researchers when the USA's Drug Enforcement Agency tried to reclassify kratom as a schedule 1 drug, which would imply it has no medical uses, and would put it in the same category as heroin and MDMA.

At present, some states in the USA have banned kratom, while others are debating doing so, which some researchers have claimed has made conducting these investigations more difficult. A number of recent research papers have discussed the potential for kratom to be employed as a harm-reduction tool for opioid use, and while we are a long way from definitive evidence, this could be a promising use of the substance, worthy of further research.

LSD

ALBERT HOFMANN, THE scientist who discovered LSD, slightly disputes the widely held story that he stumbled upon its hallucinatory effects accidentally. Hofmann was part of a programme of work at Sandoz pharmaceutical company in Basel, in north-western Switzerland, which consisted of investigating compounds that were related to naturally occurring organisms. His particular interest lay in ergot – a fungus that had previously been respon-sible for mass poisonings in the Middle Ages (known as 'St Anthony's fire'), but had recently been found to have medicinal properties as well.

In 1938, he extracted one of many lysergic acid derivatives as part of this research: lysergic acid diethylamide (LSD-25: it was the twenty-fifth derivation of ergot that Hofmann had investi-gated). After a little research on animals, it was shelved as it didn't look particularly novel or exciting to the company. But, as Hofmann describes in his autobiography, he felt 'a peculiar presen-timent – the feeling that this substance might possess properties beyond those established in the first pharmacological studies', and five years later he re-synthesised LSD in order to investigate it further.

The story goes that while synthesising it, he got some on his fingers and experienced the first LSD trip, but according to Hofmann's autobiography that's not quite what happened. He writes that he had to interrupt the end of the synthesis process as he was feeling dizzy and restless. After the weekend, he delib-erately sampled what he believed to be a tiny dose of LSD and, under the watchful eye of an assistant, proceeded to have an extreme intoxication experience – the first LSD trip.

His lab notes of the time state that he took the LSD heavily diluted in water at 4.20 p.m., started to feel dizzy and anxious at 5 p.m., and described the time between 6 and 8 p.m. as 'most severe crisis'. He believed his neighbour to be a malevolent witch, and thought that he was dying. It was also during this period that he cycled home; a bicycle ride now famous in counterculture, with bicycles often appearing on tabs of LSD, and many cele-brating Bicycle Day on 19 April in his, and LSD's, honour.

It might be hard to see the appeal of LSD from Hofmann's initial quite terrifying experience. However, even during that first trip, he saw an appeal after the initial 'horror' passed – he described 'kaleidoscopic fantastic images', and synaesthesia-like effects where everyday sounds would become moving and unique visual perceptions. People consume LSD recreationally because they want to have a 'trip', they want to experience these audio and visual hallucinations.

It's quite a different drug-taking experience than many other recreational drugs, which are often taken to enhance social experiences – although people do take LSD in groups, the experience is often very personal and inward facing. And while listening to music while on LSD might be pleasant, it's not necessarily a drug that will make you want to get up and party, although it has been associated with certain musical scenes, such as the 1960s acid psychedelia culture, and the psychedelic trance music of the 1980s.

What are the short-term effects?

If you take LSD you are in for the long haul – intoxication experiences tend to last many hours, sometimes seven, eight or even longer. LSD is generally swallowed, and is absorbed through the lining of the stomach, so the onset of intoxication is not as immediate as drugs that are snorted or injected. Intoxication will usually start around half an hour to an hour after consuming the drug, which is often taken on a tab or blotter, a small amount of liquid-diluted LSD absorbed into paper, or sometimes a sugar cube.

As well as visual and auditory hallucinations, someone tripping on LSD will likely experience distortions of time and space. Researchers have attempted to quantify the LSD intoxication experience. Studies where participants have been given LSD or placebo have found evidence that LSD alters the state of consciousness of those who take it. People experience audio-visual synaesthesia (where two senses become linked and one can cause an experience of the other), feelings of bliss, and feelings of

derealisation or depersonalisation (though these are usually positive). LSD can also influence emotional responses to experiences,
and can induce mystical experiences in some who take it.

I asked people who use LSD to attempt to describe what
intoxication feels like. Petula told me how difficult it is to explain
psychedelic intoxication to someone who has not used the drug,
stating it was 'like trying to describe a colour to a person who's
never been able to see'. Colour is something that a number of
people mentioned, from colours looking more vivid, to objects
changing colour when examined. Domingo from Little Oakley
described fabric looking like it starts to 'breathe', other people
reported this for other textured surfaces. Nature was important
to a number of people – 'trees and clouds fill me with a childlike
sense of awe'. Anika told me she limits her LSD use to during
the day, as at night 'shadows are everywhere and it feels hard to
make out where I am or what is really happening. I dislike it.'

It's very hard to overdose physically on LSD – a person would
need to take hundreds of times the usual dose to reach toxicity.
And so unlike a lot of other drugs there aren't direct physical
dangers from taking a little too much – it doesn't seem to impact
on heart rate, blood pressure or increase your likelihood of passing
out, like many other substances do.

That said, the size of the dose you take can impact on the
intensity and length of the trip you experience, so if you are
planning to use LSD, it's still far better to start with a small dose
rather than risking a larger one before you know what intoxication is like. Once you have consumed it, there's very little you
can do until the trip is over, which can take many hours.

Like a lot of drugs, the experience you will have on LSD can
be influenced by where you are, and how you are feeling when
you take it – the set and setting. But with LSD, given the
profound impact it can have on perception, misjudging this can
be particularly unpleasant. A 'bad trip' is when the perceptual
alterations experienced are negative.

One person I spoke to about their LSD experience described bad trips as occurring when she had bad feelings about the people she was with. 'It was like I could see through their poker face.' Another person told me of an 'avalanche of negative thoughts and emotions . . . but passed after ten to fifteen minutes.' 'It can really exacerbate anxiety and self-confidence issues . . . I felt like everyone knew how weird I looked . . . I felt like I might have seriously damaged my mental health and I wouldn't come back from it.'

However, a number of people were keen to point out to me that although the negative experiences might be unpleasant at the time, they welcomed the learning that the experiences brought them, some saying they did not regret having the experiences.

What are the longer-term effects?

Given that LSD has very little physical intoxication effect, it is perhaps unsurprising that it also appears to have little impact on long-term users, physically. However, there are suggestions that using LSD could impact on mental health, although whether for good or ill is harder to tell, as the evidence seems to point in both directions. Some people report improvements in psychological wellbeing. Other people find that it can bring painful emotional material to the surface, and therefore they can be psychologically agitated by using it.

It is certainly a drug not recommended for people who have a family history or high risk of mental health problems like psychosis or schizophrenia. It's not common, but LSD use has occasionally triggered mental health problems that can be long lasting.

There are links between past psychedelic use and liberal political views. Perhaps LSD causes these liberal feelings, although it's also likely that liberal people are more likely to take LSD in the first place. Interestingly, the same study found that cocaine use or alcohol use didn't predict these same liberal values. A small-scale unblinded study found long-lasting personality changes after a single dose of LSD in a lab, with people reporting the experience as being one of the most meaningful or spiritual in their lives.

LSD doesn't seem to be addictive. Which isn't to say that some people don't use it regularly. But there are some properties of LSD that mean it's not a substance that is used daily. Tolerance for the drug, where increasingly high doses are needed to feel an effect, happens quickly, and this includes cross-tolerance from other psychedelics like psilocybin (magic mushrooms). As such, if you take LSD the day after a trip, it won't really have an effect.

Lucy described herself as a regular user of LSD, and told me that meant using it around four times a year.* Partly this may be due to tolerance building up (although this is usually resolved within days rather than months), but also, as she put it, 'it's heavy stuff'. She described it as a drug that you have to prepare for, be in the right frame of mind for, put aside time for, and respect. Of course, not all people will use LSD in this way – and there is a dose-dependent effect meaning smaller doses might not be so psychologically intense as Lucy describes.

---

* This is quite different to a 'regular user' of other substances in this book – I'm a regular caffeine user, I'll use it multiple times a day. Regular smokers are also likely to use daily. Regular MDMA or cocaine use might mean monthly, regular alcohol use is likely to mean more than weekly, potentially daily.

Myths and misconceptions

LSD will make you think you can fly and you'll jump off a building

LSD is a drug that has a huge amount of mythology associated with it. Lots of these myths begun in the 1960s, where the rise in use of LSD brought about a rise in moral panic along with it. A myth often portrayed in the media is that LSD will make you think you can fly, and result in you jumping off a building or out of a window. Accidents can most certainly happen while intoxicated on LSD, due to the nature of the perceptual distortions a person can experience. But whether people are deliberately trying to fly, or rather being less careful than they usually would (similar to how people behave when intoxicated on alcohol, for example) is harder to say.

Drugs and heights do not mix – there are many instances of people intoxicated on alcohol falling from balconies or other high places, yet no one would claim that alcohol might make you think you can fly.

? PROBABLY MYTH

LSD will mess up your chromosomes

In the late 1960s, a number of high-profile research papers were published that seemed to suggest that LSD might alter or damage chromosomes – the genetic material that we each contain in every one of our cells. Papers investigating this in animals like rats, and in blood samples from humans, were published in big name journals like *Nature* and *Science*. However, a number of similar studies were also published where no such results were found.

All of these studies were really small scale, for example looking at only a handful of individuals, and some, in the case of animal studies, were giving doses of LSD far larger than humans would be likely to take. A review was published in 1971 that weighed up all the evidence from these papers, and concluded that LSD, in moderate doses, does not cause detectable genetic damage. But not before the studies that suggested harm made headlines across the USA and further afield around the world.

There was one group that the authors recommended to avoid LSD. Despite concluding that there was no strong evidence that LSD harmed unborn foetuses, the authors of the review suggested that the use of any drug during pregnancy should only occur if the benefits are strongly shown to outweigh the harms – this advice was not specific to LSD.*

✗ MYTH

LSD is stored in human fat/the spine and can be released at any time, sending you tripping unexpectedly

There are also other myths related to the body. One is that LSD gets stored in human fat, or at the base of the spine, meaning that it could be released at any time and cause an unexpected trip, or a flashback. This is nonsense; a human body will metabolise a dose of LSD within a day, and the metabolites will be excreted out in urine. And what about flashbacks themselves?

Many people will have heard urban myths of elderly people who had taken LSD in their youths suddenly having an unexpected flashback, with horrific consequences. There is some

---

* One researcher even examined the chromosomes of Timothy Leary himself. He was reportedly incredibly surprised to find that, of 200 cells examined, only two showed any chromosomal damage, and that seen was really mild. A negative finding, in a man who may have used LSD more than anyone else.

evidence to suggest that some individuals who use LSD will experience after-effects in the days and maybe even weeks following a trip. There is also a – much rarer – condition known as Hallucinogen Persisting Perception Disorder (HPPD). While there have been case reports of this happening, rarely, after one or two uses of the drug, it's more likely to happen to people who use LSD regularly over a number of years, and even then it's uncommon.

Researchers who have tried to investigate flashbacks and HPPD have tended to do so via surveys. They've found that one in around 50,000 people who use psychedelics report symptoms of HPPD that go beyond minor flashbacks and into something more disruptive to their lives, and potentially quite distressing.

✗ MYTH

LSD can wreck your mental health

What about the mind and brain? There is a widely held belief that for some people, LSD can cause schizophrenia or other severe mental health problems. And there are anecdotal reports of this, but it's challenging to research rigorously. It is the case that LSD can bring traumatic memories or thoughts to the surface, which can be extremely unpleasant, but whether this can then tip over into a serious mental disorder is harder to prove, or disprove.

As with many of these substances, it's difficult to do the research, so just because there's no evidence, doesn't mean we can be certain this isn't a risk. And given the type of experiences people can have – lights and trails across their vision, or palinopsia, the perception of an object permanently just out of view – it's a risk that shouldn't be written off.

? PARTLY TRUE

LSD will open up parts of the brain that aren't normally used

People also think that LSD can open up parts of the brain that are not usually used. I think this is related to that myth that we only use 10 per cent of our brains (and don't even get me started on that one). Certainly, people report a change in perception after using LSD, and potentially even a change in the way they think about the world, but that doesn't mean they're using more of their brain than they were previously. Having said that, new neuro-scientific evidence could suggest that the way the brain is being used might change while a person is intoxicated.

Dr Robin Carhart-Harris is the head of Psychedelic Research at Imperial College London. Along with Professor David Nutt, and a number of other colleagues, Robin has run some pioneering studies investigating how the brain works while under the influence of LSD. In one study they put twenty individuals in a Magnetic Resonance Imager (MRI) brain scanning machine – once while intoxicated, and once while not. Comparing the two brain scans for each individual, they found striking differences in functional connections across the brain. While on LSD, there was more global activity across the brain, and regions that weren't usually linked showed connections.

Obviously, this is one small-scale study, and given the perceptual alterations that happen while being intoxicated, in a way it's not surprising that there are these noticeable brain differences while intoxicated, but it is fascinating nonetheless. The authors suggest that perhaps the LSD-intoxicated brain is more similar to that of a child, where rigid or restricted thinking patterns have not yet become entrenched.

There's another widely held belief about LSD that it improves creativity. Certainly a number of creative individuals have used it, from Aldous Huxley to the Beatles, and there's even an (unsubstantiated) rumour that Kary Mullis, the Nobel prize winner, told Albert Hoffman that LSD had helped him to develop the chemical advances that would win him the Nobel. But once again we're drawn to that thorny cause-and-effect problem. Does LSD make people creative, or are creative people more drawn to seek out these types of experience?

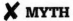 **MYTH**

Orange juice will impact on LSD intoxication

Some people believe that drinking orange juice will reduce a bad trip, while other people believe it'll enhance the intoxication experience! Clearly both can't be true. There's also another urban myth about a man on LSD believing he was an orange, or sometimes a glass of orange juice, and believed this for the rest of his life.

There's no evidence that orange juice, or vitamin C, has any effect on LSD. I don't know how this myth started, but I wonder whether it's linked to another citrus fruit – grapefruit. Individuals prescribed a variety of medications that are metabolised by a particular enzyme, the catchily titled CYP3A4, are advised not to drink grapefruit juice, because it can block the action of this enzyme and affect their action. Drugs that might be affected include certain types of statin, blood pressure drugs, anti-anxiety drugs, and a number of others.

The effects are also seen from Seville oranges, pomelos and tangelos, other citrus fruits and hybrids. There's no evidence that LSD is affected by these fruits, but it's possible something got lost in translation somewhere and an urban legend was born.

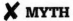 **MYTH**

Does LSD have any medical uses?

When LSD was initially discovered, and its effects were beginning to be made known, there were high hopes for it to be of use to psychiatry, in a couple of ways. Firstly, given the perceptual alterations, there was a suggestion that studying LSD intoxication could reveal secrets about mental health, given the similarities between the hallucinations and delusions of LSD, and conditions like psychosis. But researchers also wondered whether it could be used as part of psychotherapy.

Initially, in the 1950s, this was mainly to treat alcohol dependence, neurosis, and psychosomatic disorders. Early trials found evidence to support LSD-assisted therapy in reducing anxiety, depression, and pain in individuals with late-stage cancer. These studies were somewhat limited in that it is very difficult to blind such studies – it quickly becomes apparent whether a participant has been given a hallucinogen or not, and this lack of blinding can introduce bias to studies.

While some research continued over the 1980s and 1990s in Europe, particularly in Switzerland, only recently has research begun again in the USA. In 2014, researchers associated with MAPS, the Multidisciplinary Association for Psychedelic Studies, published one of the first controlled studies of LSD-assisted psychotherapy in forty years. This study was very small scale – only twelve patients with anxiety associated with life-threatening illness were recruited into the study.

They were able to blind the participants and researchers to the experimental condition of the patients by using what's known as an active placebo – a drug that also produces noticeable effects that might lead the participant or the researcher to think that the patient is in the experimental condition. In this case, they used a lower dose of LSD (20 micrograms, as compared to 200 micrograms in the experimental condition). Participants undertook two LSD (or active placebo)-assisted psychotherapy sessions. Then two months later, their anxiety was measured again.

This study was never designed to show a clinical effect – the purpose of such a small study is to investigate how well patients tolerate LSD, and to ensure there are no safety issues from administering it. The results were really positive, with participants not showing any adverse responses to LSD that persisted more than one day after treatment. They also found, twelve months after treatment, a reduction in both state- and trait-anxiety, which seemed to be sustained for twelve months.

Of course, in such a small study, we can't conclude too much. But these are tantalising results, and when considered alongside the studies on psilocybin, really might suggest a psychedelic-medicine renaissance is on the horizon. However, whether delivering such a treatment on an already overstretched health service would be possible, even if it were found to be beneficial, is another question.

Microdosing – fad or fantastic?

In recent months and years, when LSD is mentioned, if it's not a discussion of the psychedelic research detailed above, it is about microdosing. This is the concept of taking 'sub-perceptual' amounts of LSD (or other psychedelics, usually psilocybin), to improve cognition, perception, mental health, business acumen, you name it really. As yet, there are no rigorous trials into the effects of microdosing, although research is ongoing.

Qualitative research is also being undertaken, but there's a big risk of a placebo effect here. People who microdose know that they're microdosing, so while they might experience an effect, it could also be due to expectation – people expect to feel better, and so it comes to be. There's also very little consistency in how people microdose, from what amount of LSD to take, to the schedule you follow. Some people will take a tiny amount every day for a few months, others are convinced that a 'one day on, two days off' schedule is the best regimen to follow.

Quite how widespread is this behaviour is also unknown right now. For all the headlines that microdosing is endemic throughout Silicon Valley, we really have no idea how many people have tried it, for how long, and what the impact on them has been.

CHAPTER 16

MDMA

What is it? Synthetic substance first created in 1912.

Type of drug: Somewhere between a stimulant and a psychedelic, sometimes called an empathogen.

Popularity: Rose in popularity along with dance music in the 1980s and 1990s.

How consumed: Swallowed or snorted.

Timescale: Onset around half an hour, intoxication can last a few hours.

Some effects: Connection with others, euphoria, wellbeing, mild perceptual alterations, jaw clenching, increased heart rate and body temperature.

I WAS A bit too young to go to raves, and I was more of a Britpop kind of a girl myself anyway, but growing up in the 1990s I remember news reports about ecstasy, the drug young people were taking in warehouses that led them to dance until all hours. I worked out what 'Ebeneezer Goode' by the Shaman was about when I heard it on *Top of the Pops* at age nine (much to the initial shock and then amusement of my Dad, who hadn't cottoned on himself), and I very vividly remember, a few years later, the death of a young woman called Leah Betts.

This is a somewhat narrow experience of MDMA, personal to me. But it was, and remains a culturally relevant drug, being integrally linked to the clubs and raves of the 1990s, and also according to many studies more commonly used outside of these environments, in social gatherings at people's homes, for example.

Back when I first became aware of it, the talk was very much about pills, or ecstasy, and I don't think I realised for a while that ecstasy and MDMA were the same thing. Throughout the rest of this chapter, I'll refer to MDMA (this is the chemical name for the compound – 3,4-Methylenedioxymethamphetamine), but E's, ecstasy, pills, Molly, Garys . . . all these names most often refer to MDMA.

It's one of those drugs that often comes in generic tablet or powder form, so one thing to bear in mind throughout this chapter is that I'm talking about what we know about the science of the particular compound MDMA. The actual contents of a powder or pill purchased on the street may not conform to these descriptions, as substances sold as MDMA might contain no active substance, a different active substance, or could be cut with a variety of things that might impact on the severity and duration of intoxication from it.

What is it?

MDMA is a synthetic stimulant in the amphetamine family. It was first synthesised and patented in Germany in 1912, originally as an intermediate product when developing a medication to control bleeding. Its psychoactive properties weren't initially real-ised, and although there were reports of street seizures in the

USA as early as 1969, it wasn't until the mid-1970s that it began to be popularised – initially in counselling settings, particularly in California in the USA.

Chemist Alexander Shulgin synthesised it and experimented on himself – he thought that the effects would be useful within a therapeutic setting, as a related substance called MDA had been used similarly in the 1960s, so recommended it to a few therapist friends, as well as taking it recreationally himself. Its use as a recreational drug began at this time, by Shulgin himself and his friends, who apparently referred to the drug as a 'low-calorie Martini', but usage really rose when dance music became popular in Ibiza and then the UK in the mid to late 1980s.

MDMA powder is white or off-white, usually with small crystals, although larger crystals are sometimes sold as well. In tablet* form it can be any number of different shapes, sizes and colours, but generally they will look like chalky tablets. Often batches of pills will have a pattern or logo stamped into them – anything from an acid-house, yellow smiley face to a car logo.

That said, while two pills that look the same may be from the same batch, it doesn't necessarily mean they will contain the same amount of MDMA or lead to the same experience. It's also very hard to estimate how much powder is an equivalent dose to a tablet, which can lead to people accidentally taking a far higher dose than they intend to.

The criminal market around MDMA can make risks higher. Batches of tablets might be made to look the same as those with a 'reputation' of being of a certain quality, but could be completely different. Obviously, there's no standardisation or quality control in the creation of batches of MDMA, so there could be differences within the same batch, as well as between them.

---

* Although often referred to as 'pills', really MDMA comes in tablets, which are usually flat and round.

What are the short-term effects?

The intoxication effects of MDMA usually begin after around half an hour to ninety minutes if swallowed, but onset can be quicker if snorted. Intoxication can then last anywhere between four to six hours, depending on the dose consumed. Of course, there's also a lot of individual variation – this will impact on the dose that can be tolerated, the time after taking it until the effects start to be felt, how long you'll remain intoxicated before the effects wear off, that sort of thing. Your body weight, biological sex, whether or not you've eaten recently, and plain random differences will all impact on this.

Much like many other drugs, set and setting also play a part on what an intoxication experience will be like on that particular day, in that particular place, with those particular people. MDMA can be smoked, although this is an inefficient way of consuming it. It's also possible to inject it although this method of consumption is rare.

MDMA's intoxication effects made it extremely popular with clubbers, making them feel 'loved up' and connected to each other, but also energised and motivated. Feelings of euphoria are reported by people who take MDMA, and some people experience mild visual or perceptual changes. MDMA can increase feelings of wellbeing, and can enhance sensory perception (maybe that's why it can make repetitive dance music sound anthemic?).* MDMA can make people feel talkative and social, and can make people feel really connected to other people[†] – keen to talk about

---

* There's actually some evidence about why MDMA might be popular with clubbers from pharmacology research – studies have found that MDMA induces stereotypical repetitive movements in lab rats! Rat dancing?

† In the 1980s, this was so widely believed in the USA that car bumper stickers and T-shirts advised people not to get married for six weeks after taking MDMA. Timothy Leary referred to it as 'instant marriage syndrome'.

important and meaningful topics (well, they certainly seem so at the time).

Physically, MDMA is a stimulant, so it will increase heart rate and blood pressure. It can also induce jaw clenching and teeth grinding, the 'gurning' associated with clubbers who use it. You might also experience slight eye 'jiggling' (known scientifically as nystagmus).

MDMA can improve sensory perception, and can make touch more pleasurable, but if you're planning to use it to improve sexual experience this might be challenging, as it can also cause erectile dysfunction and an inability to ejaculate – for men anyway. An (admittedly small) qualitative study of heterosexual women found that the drug increased the intensity of orgasm. Surveys have also found that MDMA intoxication is associated with an increase in risk-taking behaviours related to sex as well, including having unprotected sex, multiple partners, and having sexual encounters that were later regretted.

If taken at high doses, MDMA can increase blood pressure to dangerous levels. If combined with physical exertion (like dancing, for example), high levels of MDMA can lead to hyper-thermia, the overheating of the body. This can be extremely dangerous, and can result in muscle degeneration and kidney failure. High doses of MDMA can also put a great deal of pressure on the cardiovascular system, and occasionally cause seizures.

People may take more than one dose in a single session, in an attempt to prolong the intoxication experience. However, short-term tolerance effects mean that a second dose in the same session is likely to have a shorter and possibly less pleasurable effect than the initial amount. And it will still increase the risk of overdose, so it's a hazardous strategy.

MDMA overdose can be fatal, although perhaps less commonly than media reports on MDMA deaths might suggest. UK Office of National Statistics figures from 2018 suggest that the number of deaths per year directly attributable to MDMA have ranged from fifty-eight in 2005, down to only eight in 2010, since when it has increased again. Fifty-six people had MDMA listed on their death certificate in 2017. It is also worth noting that these figures are for people who had *any* mention of MDMA on their death certificates – where only MDMA is mentioned, these numbers roughly halve.

Although very low in comparison to deaths from other substances like tobacco or alcohol, over recent years in the UK and elsewhere the number of deaths from MDMA has been going up. Although it's not known definitively why this is, some researchers believe that it could be due to factors including a lack of education about drug harms, an increase in the number of people using MDMA, and an increase in the potency of MDMA currently available to buy (or it being contaminated with more potent or dangerous substances).

What are the longer-term effects?

The longer-term effects of MDMA are far less well understood. While randomised controlled studies can be conducted to investigate the impact of intoxication while using a substance, it's not possible to assign people randomly to either use MDMA for many years or not, and so we're left to observe what people choose to do.

This creates uncertainty, as the people who use MDMA might be different from those who don't in lots of ways other than their MDMA use (for example, we know that many people who use MDMA also use a number of other psychoactive substances). And that's before we consider the impact of the illicit nature of the substance, which will make accurately estimating how much of what substance a person has used over a number of years almost impossible.

We do know a small amount from observational studies, though we need to be cautious as to how to interpret them. For example, heavy use of MDMA over prolonged periods has been linked to liver damage. There are also studies linking such patterns of use to risk of depression, anxiety, panic attacks and insomnia. It's not yet clear how clinically relevant these findings are, and it's also hard to tease out whether these are long-term risks, or related to intoxication, as acute MDMA use can also induce these symptoms.

Recent work has compiled all the research investigating associations between MDMA and executive function – the processes controlled by the brain that help us to manage tasks and achieve goals. In particular, changes in ability to perform tasks such as information updating, shifting or switching tasks, and the withholding or inhibiting of responses have been linked to MDMA use. The researchers (some of whom are now my colleagues at the University of Liverpool) then used a technique called meta-analysis to combine these papers together to assess the relationships across all the different individual studies.

This meta-analysis found that, compared to people who use other substances but not MDMA, MDMA users performed more poorly on these tasks, although the overall effect was small – the results certainly don't suggest that there are millions of people who can't function properly on a day-to-day level because of MDMA use. It's not possible to be sure that the MDMA is the cause of this difference though, as like all observational studies, the researchers could not randomly assign some people to use MDMA, and some not, so there may be other differences between users and non-users.

The use of an 'other substance-using' control group in this study is a strength, however – and just because this type of study design isn't able to work out whether an association is causal or not, that doesn't mean that the link isn't causal, only that we can't tell from this study.

Myths and misconceptions

You need to drink tonnes of water if you take MDMA

Keeping hydrated while you're intoxicated is good advice, particularly if you're dancing or somewhere really warm. But the idea that you need to drink far more water than you normally would while on MDMA came about due to the popularity of MDMA in clubs, where people were dancing for hours in hot rooms. Because MDMA can lead to hyperthermia (overheating), the need to consume water was highlighted. Clubs were encouraged to have chill-out areas and provide free water. But unfortunately, the message as to why, and in what circumstances, water should be consumed (and how much), was lost, and sometimes with tragic consequences.

Leah Betts was at a house party when she took a tablet containing MDMA in November 1995. She wasn't dancing and she wasn't in a hot room. Nonetheless, reports state that she drank seven litres of water in approximately ninety minutes,* which led to water intoxication and eventually severe swelling of the brain, which caused her to go into a coma from which she would not recover.

Another property of MDMA is that it can reduce the ability to urinate. This property can make the drinking of vast amounts of water even more dangerous. At the inquest into her death, toxicologist John Henry is reported as saying, 'If Leah had taken the drug alone, she might well have survived. If she had drunk the amount of water alone, she would have survived.' It's extremely unlikely that Leah would have consumed so much water if she hadn't taken MDMA – the actions of people while

---

* Advice states that a person should sip approximately one litre of water in the course of an hour if they are dancing, and less if they are not.

intoxicated are important to consider, as well as toxicity from the substance itself.

? PARTLY TRUE

MDMA causes brain lesions

It seems likely that this myth may have resulted from a since-retracted paper. Researchers at Johns Hopkins University in the USA injected five squirrel monkeys, and five baboons with three moderate doses of what they believed to be MDMA, and found impact on levels of the neurotransmitters dopamine and serotonin in the animals. Their findings were published in the journal *Science*, one of the most highly respected scientific journals in the world, and in their paper they concluded that their results should concern recreational MDMA users, who might be 'unwittingly putting themselves at risk . . . of neuropsychiatric disorders'.

At the time this finding was extremely surprising, as MDMA had not been linked to an impact on dopamine before, but this study suggested not only dopaminergic neurotoxicity, but also found that the animals in the study displayed symptoms related to Parkinson's disease. But all was not as it seemed. Almost exactly a year after the paper was published, the authors retracted it. After they had tried and failed to replicate the study, they began to grow suspicious that something had gone awry in their original study.

Although the MDMA batch that they used for the initial study had since run out, by examining the brains of the monkeys and baboons in the study, they worked out that in fact they had administered the primates methamphetamine, and not MDMA at all. At the doses they had given, their findings were much more as expected from methamphetamine, and the authors duly retracted the paper. But not before the initial findings received a great deal of media attention. Not only that, but the study didn't find 'brain lesions' in the first place – pictures used to illustrate the study in the media used brain images that appeared to have holes in them, but in fact the image showed differences in blood flow in different regions, not holes at all.

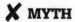 **MYTH**

MDMA (powder) is safer than ecstasy (tablets), because it's not cut with other things

Not true. While tablets are often cut with anything from caffeine to amphetamine, it is perfectly possible for a powder to be mixed with these substances as well, and samples have been found that contain synthetic cathinones (such as mephedrone), or other substances such as PMA that have been found in both tablets and powder – some of which might be more harmful than MDMA at the same, or even at smaller doses.

✗ MYTH

Does MDMA have any medical uses?

Experiments are ongoing in trying to use low doses of MDMA during therapy sessions to help people with post-traumatic stress disorder talk about their trauma in an environment that doesn't trigger their panic. Because the intoxication effects of MDMA can make an individual feel safe, connected with those around them and motivated, it may aid the treatment of PTSD, which is notoriously hard, as often talking about the traumatic event can trigger a panic response. At present results are thin on the ground, and largely conducted by a small group of researchers, but promising. It will be really interesting to see whether other independent groups replicate these findings.

Some researchers believe that chronic MDMA use leads to serotonin depletion over time. This has been seen in primate research, but is harder to assess in humans. A recent study meta-analysed the existing work where molecular-imaging brain scans of humans had been carried out. They found seven studies that had assessed this, and the evidence suggested a reduction in the numbers of serotonin transporter – a protein that controls how the neurotransmitter passes information between neurons – in ecstasy users compared to drug-using controls. Again though, as levels were not measured before the use of MDMA, it's not certain these differences weren't there before.

Of course, this doesn't mean that MDMA is not harmful to serotonin levels in the brain. And it's also not known whether, if this is the case, this depletion is reversible or not. As with so many illicit drugs, carrying out this research is tricky, relies on self-report, and is not ethical or practical to investigate via randomised trials; so it is often done by observing what people choose to do, thus not being able to rule out other differences. Even if we don't know for sure, it's certainly good advice to avoid taking any substance too regularly, keep doses low, and allow plenty of sober time between intoxication events.

CHAPTER 17

Nitrous Oxide

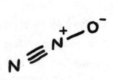

What is it? A gas inhaled for its short-lasting head rush.
Type of drug: Anaesthetic.
Popularity: Popular in the UK and Netherlands in
  particular.
How consumed: Inhaled, usually from party balloons.
Timescale: Very short – intoxication lasts only as long as you
  breathe the substance in.
Some effects: Euphoria, slight dissociation, dizziness, nausea,
  loss of fine motor function, headaches.

DESPITE IT SEEMING like a relatively modern concern, popular
with young people at the moment, nitrous oxide – and even
recreational nitrous-oxide use – has been around for quite a while.
In the 1800s, not long after its discovery, nitrous oxide was
somewhat of a party trick in Georgian Britain. And that was
largely due to Sir Humphry Davy – the Cornish chemist and
inventor, who was a lecturer at the hugely popular Royal

Institution in London, and would go on to become President of the Royal Society.

He promoted and demonstrated its effects via lectures, pamphlets and even books. The gas would be handed round at highbrow gatherings, and London theatres even put on 'Laughing Gas' evenings, where members of the public could queue up to try it.

What is it?

Nitrous oxide is a molecule made up of one oxygen and two nitrogen atoms. At room temperature, it is a colourless, slightly sweet-tasting gas. Nitrous oxide is used extensively in the catering industry, as a pressurised gas to whip cream, and is used in medicine as an anaesthetic and sedative. But nitrous is also popular as a recreational drug – its popularity evidenced by the number of 'whippits' – small metal canisters containing the gas – found discarded in the streets of UK cities (certainly Bristol and Liverpool, where I've lived recently).

The statistics back this up – it's more popular as a recreational drug in the UK than in the rest of the world. In 2018, the Global Drug Survey found that 14.1 per cent of people who responded to their survey reported ever using nitrous, with nearly 7 per cent having done so in the past year. These numbers were even higher when just looking at the UK. The only country where nitrous is more popular than the UK is the Netherlands.

This popularity may be due to the ease with which it can be obtained. Nitrous canisters can be placed in metal dispensers (sometimes referred to as 'crackers') that release the pressurised gas. Party balloons are filled with the gas and inhaled.

What are the short-term effects?

Nitrous intoxication is extremely short-term – if you stop breathing in the gas, you stop feeling the effect almost immediately. The sensations that people intoxicated on nitrous report are euphoria, and potentially a slight feeling of disconnection from themselves. Nitrous can induce dizziness, so people using it are at risk of falling over. In rare circumstances, people can risk asphyxiation if they are inhaling the gas with their mouth and nose covered and they pass out.

It can also make individuals feel nauseous. Headaches are a commonly reported after-effect of a heavy session using nitrous. The gas can also impact on a person's ability to perform fine motor functions (like writing a text message), and this can persist for perhaps fifteen minutes after they stop inhaling it.

Individuals are at substantially more risk of harm if they inhale the gas directly out of the dispenser. Not only is inhaling pressurised gas directly into your face extremely dangerous, but there is further peril, because when the pressurised gas is released, it is at an extremely cold temperature. People who inhale direct from the dispenser can risk severe damage to their mouths and even their larynx or lungs, including frostbite.

When used in a medical setting, nitrous is always administered with oxygen included in the gaseous mix. When recreational drug users fill a balloon with whipped cream propellant, this isn't the case. As such, there's an increased risk of hypoxia – a lack of oxygen reaching the tissues in the body. This can be highly dangerous, as if oxygen isn't reaching important organs like the brain or liver, damage can be done to them within minutes.

What are the longer-term effects?

Although nitrous has relatively low toxicity, and many people therefore believe it's a safe drug, regular use of nitrous oxide can lead to longer-term and in some cases quite serious risks. There's some suggestion that it can be dependence forming, although this is based on case studies rather than longitudinal studies, so whether this is a large risk or not is unclear.

A growing concern in populations who regularly use nitrous is vitamin B12 deficiency. The nitrous interacts with the vitamin B12 molecule, which impairs it from functioning in the body. Mild symptoms of low vitamin B12 can include tingling in fingers and toes, numbness, and difficulty walking. In extreme cases this deficiency can cause anaemia, as well as impacting on the brain and cognitive ability, potentially even causing depression and dementia.

There have been case studies of spinal-cord degeneration reported in the past couple of years, which have been linked to recreational nitrous use, and there's some suggestion that the impact on vitamin B12 leads to damage to the fatty myelin sheaths that surround neurons (cells found in the brain and the spinal cord). The myelin surrounding neurons is essential for enabling electrical impulses to pass quickly along the length of neurons, some of which are over a metre long.

Although the rates of low vitamin B12 symptoms in nitrous users are not well documented, this is an important risk that people using nitrous need to be aware of, so they can monitor their usage and ensure they are not using so much that they become B12 deficient. Some users report taking vitamin supplements if they are using very heavily, but whether this would improve their levels is unclear. When the individuals in these case studies were asked about their use, they on average reported using nitrous two or three times a week, at high levels (some reported using over 100 whippets on a given day).

Nitrous oxide is teratogenic. This means it is a drug that can disturb or disrupt the development of an embryo or foetus. Women who are pregnant – or think they might be – may not be aware that this is the case, and risk damaging their unborn child if they use nitrous while pregnant.

Myths and misconceptions

Hippie crack is more dangerous than laughing gas

Hippie crack is just another name for nitrous oxide – so there's no difference in risk of using, because it's the same substance. However, the name 'hippie crack' is potentially misleading. Nitrous oxide is a greenhouse gas, and therefore individuals who want to save the planet and reduce the negative impact that climate change is having on our environment should probably think twice before accepting a balloon at a party (although admittedly the amount used recreationally pales in comparison to that generated by the use of fertilisers).

Regarding the safety; although deaths from nitrous are rare, they're not unheard of. In the UK, Office for National Statistics figures indicate that in recent years nitrous was involved in a handful of deaths every year.

 MYTH

Nitrous causes intoxication by starving the brain of oxygen

When nitrous is inhaled without oxygen, the risk of hypoxia, where the brain can be starved of oxygen, is increased. However, this isn't what causes nitrous to have the effects that recreational users seek. If it was, maybe we could all simply hold our breath and get the same effect? When nitrous is administered in a medical setting, the ratio of gas to oxygen is required to be fifty-fifty, to minimise the risk of hypoxia, as it can be extremely dangerous, as detailed above.

✗ MYTH

Does nitrous oxide have medical uses?

The short answer to this is yes, nitrous oxide was one of the first anaesthetics. However, it has a rather unusual, and slightly sad, history in terms of its medical use. It was discovered in the 1770s by Joseph Priestley, after he heated iron filings soaked in nitric acid. He inhaled some of the resultant 'nitrous, or dephlo-gisticated airs' as he put it, and noticed feeling giddy and less sensitive to pain.

A few years later, in the 1790s, the Pneumatic Institution was set up in Clifton, the leafy area of Bristol in the south-west of England, to further research gases that were being discovered and whether they might have medical benefits. It was here that Humphrey Davy first encountered nitrous oxide – and after testing it on himself, he quickly came to refer to it as 'laughing gas'. He initially believed the gas might be useful to treat tuber-culosis, but in his 1800 book on the gas, he highlights that it could probably 'be used with great advantage during surgical operations'.

It's here the story of nitrous oxide takes a slightly unusual, and quite upsetting, detour. Despite this being a time in history without any safe anaesthetics, it took nearly fifty years for nitrous to become widely used in this way. In the meantime, it became extremely popular as a fairground attraction, or for use at laughing-gas parties, a favourite with the British upper classes.

A few individuals on both sides of the Atlantic tried to promote the use of nitrous as an anaesthetic during this time, but perhaps due to its image as a recreational drug, were not taken seriously. Probably the best known of these is Horace Wells, a dentist from Connecticut, USA. He attended a demonstration of nitrous and noticed a man under the influence of the gas accidentally injure himself – without pain. He and a colleague began to use the gas in their dentistry, and found it to reduce or eliminate pain in their patients.

He took his findings to Massachusetts General Hospital at Harvard University, and gave a demonstration. While it was a partial success, it seems probable that the dose or duration of supply was incorrect in this instance, and the patient reportedly cried out. Wells was ridiculed, called a fraud, and ultimately not taken seriously. He took his own life a few years later.

A remarkably similar story happened in England at around this time. A young doctor called Henry Hill Hickman experimented with the use of nitrous for anaesthesia on animals – and believed it could revolutionise human surgery. He presented his idea in both England and France, going to speak to the Royal Academy of Medicine in Paris, but he was not taken seriously. His early death at twenty-nine years of age prevented him from pursuing the idea further.

Eventually interest in the use of nitrous was rekindled, particularly after the rise in popularity of chloroform and ether, and the high risk of overdose from them. Once techniques were developed to allow the administration of nitrous alongside oxygen, the use of the gas as an anaesthetic, analgesic and tranquiliser became more popular.

These days, nitrous is less widely used in everyday anaesthesia, mostly because it can cause nausea, which people report as unpleasant. However, it does have uses as what is known as a 'carrier' gas. It's not able to induce general anaesthesia by itself, but if it is combined with another anaesthetic it can aid the uptake of the other gas and deepen its effect. It means less of the other anaesthetic is required to achieve the same result.

It's still used in obstetric practice – you've probably heard of 'gas and air' being given to pregnant women to help with pain during childbirth. This might make it sound perfectly safe, but there are a number of mechanisms in place to ensure that it doesn't cause harm, even in this controlled environment, with medical supervision readily on hand. Women are given a device to allow them to self-administer the gas with an 'on demand valve'. This means that should they inhale too much gas and fall unconscious, the valve will be released and the supply of gas will stop. A couple of breaths of air and a person will no longer feel the effects of the drug.

Nitrous can also be useful in Accident and Emergency departments. A person can take a few breaths of nitrous-and-oxygen, and potentially have a dislocated arm re-inserted without pain or distress, as it causes sedation and pain relief.

What don't we know?

Given nitrous was discovered in the 1700s, it's quite surprising how little we still know about how it works, and anaesthetics in general. This brings us to the so-called 'hard problem' of consciousness. How and why do we experience consciousness, and how does it manifest in our bodies? In his excellent TED talk, neuroscientist Anil Seth describes his experience of going under due to anaesthesia as feeling akin to 'ceasing to exist'. He defines it as distinct from sleeping, as when you awake from a sleep you have a sense of time having passed, while this isn't the case when waking from anaesthesia.

We don't understand the link between our physical brains and our mental states anywhere near well enough, and as such, it is hard for us to understand how drugs that impact on consciousness cause this effect. Whole books have been written about this, from both philosophical and scientific perspectives, but I'm afraid they don't, and I certainly don't, have the answers just yet. Anil Seth uses his TED talk to propose that all of our perception is a controlled hallucination – but there's still a way to go before the hard problem is solved.

Focus on: Psychedelics

The term 'psychedelic' was believed to have been coined by a psychiatrist called Humphrey Osmond, and is from the Greek words *'psyche'* meaning mind and *'deloun'* meaning 'to reveal or make visible'. So the term psychedelic means soul-revealing or mind-manifesting. Psychedelic drugs are those that alter perceptions – visual changes, or changes in the ability to perceive time are common.

Which drugs are psychedelics?

LSD, magic mushrooms (psilocybin is the active compound here), mescaline (found in cacti), DMT, 2-CB and a whole host of less common synthetic substances related to it are all classed as psychedelics. Salvia is sometimes considered a psychedelic due to its perception-altering qualities, but chemically it is quite different to these others.

At a molecular level, there are two different types of psychedelics – drugs that cause a perceptual-altering or 'mind-manifesting' (as the term psychedelic means) effect – tryptamines and phenethylamines. Simple tryptamine molecules (in particular DMT) very closely resemble the molecular structure of serotonin, a neurotransmitter found throughout our brains and bodies. Psilocybin, LSD and DMT are all tryptamines.

The other class of psychedelics is phenethylamines. This includes mescaline and synthetic psychedelics such as 2-CB, DOM and 2C-T-7, although it also includes a number of other substances you'll find throughout this book, including MDMA and amphetamine, and also the neurotransmitter dopamine.

What effects do psychedelics have?

The key features of psychedelics are that they alter perception. Psychedelic intoxication is often associated with kaleidoscopic artwork, patterns repeating and folding in on themselves, and colours exploding off the page in a vivid rainbow. Sounds and vision can become linked, akin to synaesthesia, where senses are connected. Perceptions of time and space can also become distorted at higher doses. Patterns, when looked at, can appear to pulse or move about. Depending on the type of psychedelic, hallucinations can replace what is really there, or sit superimposed on top of 'normal' vision.

Psychedelics can also impact on mood and emotion. This can happen both during intoxication, and potentially following it. Some people who use psychedelics do so because they believe it will change their perspective about their lives. A number of psychedelics including psilocybin are being investigated as potential treatments for mental health problems such as depression.

Psychedelics do not tend to be dependence forming (although it's not impossible to develop problematic use of psychedelics). People who use psychedelics tend to do so sporadically – regular use of a psychedelic might mean using it once every month or two. If you take a psychedelic immediately after a previous dose, the second dose will have no effect, as tolerance to the substance builds up quickly.

There's some evidence that psychedelics are unsafe for people who have a high risk of mental health problems such as psychosis – a psychedelic trip could trigger a psychotic episode in people vulnerable to them.

CHAPTER 18

PCP: Angel Dust

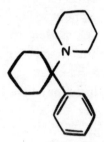

PHENCYCLIDINE, OFTEN CALLED PCP or angel dust, was initially developed as a dissociative anaesthetic, back in the 1920s. It was tested extensively in human participants, but its risk of severe side-effects led researchers to develop a similar compound with fewer side-effects (that substance was ketamine). PCP is quite a challenging substance to write about because it can be taken in a load of different ways, can have very varied effects, and although it has been studied extensively as an anaesthetic, how it is used recreationally has been less well documented.

As well as that, it is a substance that has had a lot written about it in the press throughout its history. The drug has been demonised and linked to superhuman strength, cannibalistic tendencies, and horrific attacks and murders. But exaggeration and misinformation can certainly occur around illicit drugs – so exactly how much of its bad reputation does PCP deserve? I've done my best to cut through all the hyperbole and present what we know, while making it clear what we don't, and what's incorrect.

What are the short-term effects?

PCP can be taken in many different ways – as an oil, a liquid, a powder, crystals or in tablet form. PCP oil is yellowish in colour, while powders, crystals or tablets can range in colour from white to light brown. As well as coming in multiple guises, PCP can also be consumed in a variety of ways, including sniffing, swallowing, injecting or smoking (some people will spray PCP onto tobacco or cannabis and smoke it like a cigarette). Smoking PCP in this way is sometimes called 'getting wet' or referred to as 'embalming fluid'.

The method of consumption will impact on the timings of intoxication experience. Smoking or injecting will lead to a faster intoxication onset (around two minutes) than swallowing (half an hour to an hour), with sniffing being somewhere between the two. Reports of how long intoxication lasts are extremely varied. Some say a person will remain intoxicated for two to five hours, some say four to eight, others suggest it could last for as long as forty-eight hours. Length of intoxication could also be affected by a number of things – route of administration or size of dose, as well as various factors about the person themselves.

When a person takes PCP, it's very hard to predict what their intoxication experience will be like. The dissociative effect can induce a numbing, dream-like or floaty sensation. Some can experience audio or visual hallucinations, and alterations in time perception, where it could speed up or slow down. PCP can alter mood, and can make someone feel detached from reality. For some this could be severe, in the form of paranoia or even transient psychotic experiences. If people are already prone to psychosis, PCP can make their condition substantially worse. Physiologically, PCP will increase body temperature, heart rate and blood pressure, and it might make you constipated.

At very high doses a person will experience the anaesthetic effects of the substance – a person's breathing can become slow and shallow, although some people find that PCP causes irregular breathing, where breathing will be fast and then stop briefly before starting again. Some people can experience convulsions after taking PCP. It can cause uncontrollable eye movements, and the anaesthetic properties can also mean that a person on PCP can hurt themselves quite severely without realising.

More contentious is whether PCP can cause aggression and violence. Certainly, when PCP was a popular* recreational drug in the USA in the 1990s, media reports suggested it could make people extremely aggressive. These reports also stated that PCP gave people superhuman strength (more on that later). PCP intoxication has been linked to suicide. Again, it's not necessarily clear whether PCP causes this directly, or whether people are more prone to take risks or have accidents while intoxicated.

That's quite a list of effects. Some seem stimulant-like, some

---

* Although how popular it was may have been exaggerated, as described later in the chapter.

depressant-like, some hallucinogenic, and some analgesic. As I've said above, it's extremely difficult to predict whether PCP will make a person sleepy or super-energised, whether it'll increase their heart rate and blood pressure, or slow their breathing. Similar to alcohol, it's been found that PCP impacts on loads of different neurotransmitters throughout the brain – NMDA, GABA, dopamine, serotonin, norepinephrine, opioid receptors. All of these receptors and neurotransmitters are involved in different brain functions, which might explain the wide variety of effects, some of which seem contradictory.

PCP is also soluble in fats, water and alcohol, and this might explain why the effects can be so different from person to person. All sorts of things might impact on what kind of PCP intoxication experience a person has – biological sex, height and weight, what a person has eaten, whether they've had alcohol, and general health will all impact on how and where PCP is absorbed by the body, so the intoxication effects can vary wildly.

Taking too much PCP can be extremely dangerous, with a risk of hyperthermia, coma and death. PCP can also have some pretty unpleasant withdrawal symptoms if a person stops taking it after using it for a while. These can include psychotic experiences, anxiety, tremors, diarrhoea and eye shakes.

What are the longer-term effects?

Longer term, there's evidence that regular heavy use of PCP can lead to tolerance and dependence, meaning higher doses will be required to get the same effect, and potentially the wish to take the substance could turn into a need. Heavy use has been associated with later memory problems, depression, psychosis and paranoia, as well as poor appetite and weight loss. Whether this is due to the substance itself, or the impact it has on a person's ability to take good care of themselves in terms of sleep, nutrition and the like is harder to say, but either way the outcome on the individual remains.

Myths and misconceptions

PCP is a substance that got a whole lot of media attention, particularly in the 1990s. As such, myths and misconceptions built up around it. Here are some of them.

PCP will give you superhuman strength

In 1991, in Los Angeles, after a car chase, police officers were caught on film using what appeared to be excessive force to restrain a man named Rodney King. King's injuries included broken bones and multiple bruises and lacerations. It was deemed to be severe enough to warrant the police officers involved having to face prosecution for it, and the trial had plenty of media coverage.

The police officers' defence stated that King appeared to be intoxicated on PCP. They said he was able to stand even while police officers tried to 'swarm' him to restrain him, and that he continued to try and get up after he had been hit and restrained multiple times. At the time, it was often reported that PCP would give people superhuman strength, and indeed police officers in LA at the time had been instructed that they could be harmed by people who were intoxicated on PCP because of this.

In actual fact, there's no evidence that PCP can give an individual superhuman strength. What it might do is remove a person's restraint, and numb them to any pain, which might make them less inhibited and therefore appear stronger. Even this is speculation though, it could also be that given PCP was used mostly by black men in their twenties, this profiling of PCP users as dangerous violent superhumans could very well have been tinged with more than a little racism.

As for Rodney King, he admitted to being intoxicated on alcohol (which he claimed was why he fled from the police in the first place), but denied having taken PCP, and an expert witness toxicologist testified that alcohol and cannabis were found in his blood sample, but PCP was not.

 MYTH

PCP will turn you into a cannibal

The proliferation of this myth is likely linked to the case of a rapper called Big Lurch. In 2002 he killed his roommate, cut her open, and apparently ate some of her lung. There are also cases of people gouging their own eyes out while on PCP, of people walking into traffic, and many many pages of press coverage over the years have been filled with accusations of PCP-induced murder and mayhem. Is this right?

The effect that PCP will have on someone will depend on their underlying personality, their current psychological state, the environment that they are in when they take it, and any other underlying risk factors for severe mental health problems like schizophrenia.* It's highly unlikely that one-off use of PCP in an individual with no risk factors for psychosis would lead to an extreme event like the ones detailed in the media.

Which isn't to detract from the risks to the self and to others from intoxication, and the possibility for awful consequences when a person does develop psychosis after taking a substance.

---

* And even with severe illnesses like schizophrenia, this does not mean a person is therefore more likely to become violent. In fact, lots of research suggests that people with schizophrenia are more likely to be a danger to themselves than to other people. Some research has even found that they are also more likely to be the victims of crime, which might indicate some sort of confounding going on in this research.

But the substance does not exist in isolation, and therefore the risks of a reaction like that of Big Lurch, whether he was on PCP or not, will depend on all sorts of things. Set and setting, as we've seen throughout this book, can't be underestimated.

✗ **MYTH**

Does PCP have any medical uses?

PCP was initially developed by a pharmaceutical company, and tested on a number of different animals in order to ascertain its properties. Right from the outset, it was clear that PCP was unpredictable. It had quite different effects in different animals. In rodents it seemed to cause 'excited drunken' behaviour, while in pigeons it induced what researchers referred to as a 'cataleptoid immobilised state'. In dogs, it cause delirium. When tested on monkeys, it showed enough promise as an anaesthetic to warrant testing in humans.

It was found to be safe as an anaesthetic, but participants given it in trials reported unusual and unpleasant side-effects during recovery, some of which included feelings of sensory deprivation, like being unable to feel their limbs. Its use in humans as an anaesthetic was halted, and chemists continued to tweak the chemical formula, looking for a similar anaesthetic without such extreme side-effects (and discovering ketamine in the process). But this wasn't completely the end for PCP's use in medicine.

Some researchers noticed that the intoxication effects of PCP looked quite similar to symptoms in patients with schizophrenia, and wondered whether this similarity could be harnessed in some way. Researchers at the Lafayette clinic in Michigan began a programme of work where they compared the effect of PCP intoxication in healthy individuals with the behaviour of patients with schizophrenia. They even added a third and fourth condition, LSD or barbiturate intoxication, as control groups in their studies.

They ran a battery of tests on different types of abilities, including things like attention and reaction time, and found that people on PCP performed more similarly to people with schizophrenia across the tasks, as compared to either those sedated by a barbiturate or those intoxicated on LSD. Interestingly, they found that people given PCP tolerated the drug better when in conditions of sensory isolation than when not isolated. The researchers reported that they used this finding to inform their practice with their patients with schizophrenia, allowing them space and isolation, and, anecdotally at least, seeing improvements in symptoms after doing this.

Research into schizophrenia using PCP was also conducted in animals. Since it was hypothesised that PCP could induce an experience like schizophrenia, pharmacologists could test the potential effects of drugs being developed for treating schizophrenia by seeing whether those drugs could reverse the effects of PCP. This tended to occur in the 1950s and 1960s, when little was understood both about the effects of PCP and schizophrenia. These days it is now accepted that although PCP might be similar to some aspects of schizophrenia, it does not operate in exactly the same way, and therefore is probably quite a limited model of the disease.

We are still a long way from discovering all there is to know about schizophrenia, in fact many people argue that the set of symptoms of the disease are so varied that in all likelihood it may not be one disease, and that we should move away from the diagnosis entirely. Whatever we call it, it can be a debilitating and life-changing diagnosis to receive, and therefore substances that can induce psychosis, even if transiently, should be taken seriously.

How popular is PCP?

Despite media reports, PCP has never been one of the more popular recreational drugs, probably because the intoxication effect can be extreme. Its use has been best documented in the USA, and reports suggest that patterns of use have tended to be localised into various metropolitan areas across the country. A recent study looked at hospital admissions for PCP intoxication in the USA between the 1970s and the early 2010s. They found a waxing and waning pattern, which they suggested could be due to 'generational forgetting'. When PCP is more widely used, its effects are better known, and its popularity decreases, and when a new generation who don't know its effects come along, its popularity increases again.

That could be an explanation for this, but there could be any number of other explanations, too. For example, rising or falling hospital admissions could be due to quality and strength of the substance at the time, which could be affected by all sorts of things. It's very hard to say. It's also worth noting that hospital admissions are a very extreme example of use. If you've had to go to hospital, you're necessarily having a bad time, but this might not be true of all users.

Similarly, it's rare for people to have used only one substance. One research paper looking at hospital admissions for PCP use found that one in four people admitted had also taken benzodiazepines, 40 per cent had also consumed cannabis, and 40 per cent had alcohol in their system as well.

CHAPTER 19

Poppers: Alkyl Nitrites

AMYL NITRITE

What is it? Originally a treatment for angina, now used to improve sex.
Type of drug: Volatile solvent-smelling liquid.
Popularity: Popular in certain scenes or circles.
How consumed: Inhaled, from a cloth or straight from the bottle.
Timescale: Short lasting – 2 to 5 minutes.
Some effects: Headrush, relaxation of smooth muscle, warmth, headache, sweating, skin flush.

'POPPERS' IS A colloquial term for a group of substances called alkyl nitrites. Amyl nitrite is probably the best known of these, but others are called cyclohexyl nitrite, isobutyl nitrite, isopropyl nitrite, and butyl nitrite.

Amyl nitrite was originally synthesised way back in 1844, by a French chemist called Antoine Jérôme Balard. It was created and marketed as a treatment for angina, because the expansion of blood vessels that it induced can lower blood pressure and improve blood flow to the heart.* This is also how they got their name. The liquid was purchased in 'single serve' capsules or ampoules, which the user cracked or 'popped' to release the vapour to inhale. Poppers were reportedly used in high numbers by soldiers during the Vietnam War.

Historian Ian Young, in his book *The Stonewall Experiment*, suggests that poppers were heavily marketed at the gay community, with adverts in gay magazines in the USA and in the UK in the 1960s and 1970s. There are even some reports that gay clubs would pump amyl nitrite into the air in clubs, over the heads of people dancing, although this could be an urban myth.

These day poppers are found as liquids, usually sold in small bottles with brightly coloured labels and ridiculous names like Bang Aroma, Zap or Rock Hard (the reason for this one might become apparent later). It's currently legal to sell alkyl nitrites in many countries around the world – as long as they're marketed as not for human consumption. Often they are sold euphemistically as deodorisers or leather cleaners, sometimes in sex shops or online.

These names and locations of sale might give a hint as to some of the appeal of poppers, and the groups of people who might use them. The effects of poppers (discussed in more detail below) make them appealing as something to aid or augment sex – they can enhance intensity and length of orgasm for some people. But poppers are also used in other settings – they were particularly associated with certain music scenes including disco and rave, particularly the gay disco scene in the 1970s.

For those, like me, who are children of the 1990s, you might also be aware of the (excellent) Suede song 'Animal Nitrate'. In

---

* Though, it goes without saying, self-prescribing yourself poppers if you have heart problems is an extremely bad idea, and we have better and more effective medications now – go and see a doctor.

all likelihood this is a reference to poppers, although it is 'nitrate' rather than 'nitrite' – which is chemically slightly different. Perhaps Brett Anderson was deliberately being a little coy with the reference, and it certainly got under some radars, being played on the radio and performed at the 1993 Brit Awards, which had nationwide TV coverage.

What are the short-term effects?

At room temperature the strong solvent-smelling liquid becomes a vapour, and people can inhale it. Most commonly, it is inhaled straight from the bottle, although some individuals will transfer some to a cloth or cotton wool to inhale from, and there are reports that some people will dip the end of an unlit cigarette into the liquid then inhale it through the other end.*

If they do, they will likely experience an immediate onset and very short-term intoxication experience, often no more than two to five minutes in total. This mainly consists of a headrush – a feeling of lightheadedness, dizziness and a throbbing head.

Poppers relax the smooth muscle throughout the body. Smooth muscles are those in areas of the body where an elastic effect is required. This includes muscles that run alongside blood vessels, and relaxation of these muscles means that these vessels will widen and blood pressure will drop. Smooth muscle also includes sphincters and the muscles in the anus and vagina walls, which is why it is used by people when they are having sex.

Poppers can induce feelings of warmth. Less pleasant effects include headache, sweating, increased heart rate, and skin flush in some people. Despite their common use during sex, some

---

* If you inhale poppers in this way, it's extremely important a) to inhale from the opposite end to the one that you dipped, and b) not to light the cigarette afterwards, as alkyl nitrites are extremely flammable.

men report erectile problems after using poppers. The liquid itself can give chemical burns if it touches the skin – and it's extremely dangerous if swallowed. It can cause organ failure, blindness, unconsciousness, coma and brain damage, and people have been known to die after swallowing it. If you or someone you know has swallowed it, go to hospital immediately. People have also died after inhaling very large quantities of poppers – particularly if they're blocking their airways and are unable to take on oxygen.

What are the longer-term effects?

Harms from poppers are fairly rare, but when they do occur, they can be serious. Poppers can increase risks of harm in people with blood pressure or heart problems. It's also more high-risk to take poppers if you're on blood-pressure medication, or if you've taken Viagra. Both Viagra and poppers can lower the blood pressure, and if both are taken at the same time this can be really dangerous, reducing blood flow to the brain and other vital organs, and potentially leading to stroke or death.

Although this is rare, the Office for National Statistics report that between 2001 and 2016 alkyl nitrites were mentioned on the death certificates of eighteen individuals, making up 3 per cent of deaths related to volatile substances over that fifteen-year period. If people are regularly sniffing poppers straight from the bottle, the repeated minor contact around the nose or mouth can lead to crusty skin in those areas. Inhaling, particularly through the mouth, can also lead to accidental aspiration of the liquid into the lungs, rather than the vapour. This can also be dangerous and medical assistance should be sought if this occurs.

Some medical case studies of people who have used poppers heavily have found maculopathy – a type of eye damage, or temporary damage to the retina or foevea, which is seemingly reversible after a person stops using. But it's hard to extrapolate from case studies, and there haven't been any studies that have investigated the links between poppers and eye damage on a larger scale.

Heavy regular use of poppers has also been linked to an increased risk of methaemoglobinaemia, where the body is starved of oxygen due to a change in haemoglobin, the substance in blood that transports oxygen around the body to our cells. Some reports suggest this condition even turns the blood a 'chocolate brown' colour. Unfortunately, it's unclear how much is too much in this case. But as with all substances, it's always sensible to have regular breaks where the substance is not used, to allow your body to recover.

Although there's little evidence to suggest that poppers are addictive, tolerance may build up if they are used repeatedly over a short period of time, which is another reason that regular breaks from using them are a good idea.

Myths and misconceptions

Poppers increase the risk of cancer

Back in the 1980s, a research paper was published that reported a link between the use of poppers among gay men, and the risk of a rare cancer of the blood vessels called Kaposi's sarcoma. This cancer is opportunistic, which means it can affect people whose immune systems are already compromised, for example if they are HIV positive. The researchers looked at lifestyle behaviours that predicted a likelihood to develop this cancer, compared to likelihood to develop other diseases such as pneumonia, and found that regular heavy use of poppers predicted Kaposi's.

Many studies have found that heavy use of poppers is correlated with an inclination to partake in risky sexual behaviours, and also an increased risk of contracting HIV, among men who have sex with men. But this isn't to say that the poppers cause the increase in risk. The relationship may well be in the other direction – people who are more likely to take risks when having sex might therefore be more likely to use poppers as well. Either way, given the association between the two, perhaps it's not surprising that this rare cancer shown to be linked to having HIV is also associated with using poppers, if contracting HIV is associated with it.

It's really important to make this point – poppers weren't causing people to develop AIDS – because back in the 1980s when people, but in particular gay and bisexual men, were first becoming ill with AIDS, poppers were pointed to as a potential cause of what was initially called 'gay cancer'. It was, in all probability, a vilification of homosexuality as deviant behaviour, painting it as men having drug-fuelled sex leading to the illness.

More recently the link between poppers and cancer has been looked into again, using a large-scale study of people with and without HIV across the USA, called the multicenter AIDS cohort study (MACS). MACS has been running for over thirty years, and has around 7,000 participants. Using this dataset, researchers found no association between use of poppers and risk of a variety of virus-based cancers across their sample.

However, in a sub-sample of men without HIV, who were aged between fifty and seventy years old, they did find evidence of a link between heavy poppers use and a risk of virus-driven cancers, caused by things like exposure to HPV (human papillomavirus – the same virus that can cause cervical cancer). This is quite a specific sub-sample of their analysis, and the same pattern was not seen in men of the same age who did have a diagnosis of HIV, which makes it even harder to interpret.

It may be that poppers might temporarily lower a person's immune system, which combined with risky sexual behaviours that could expose a person to viruses (like HPV for example) that increase the risk of cancer. But this is a long way from definitive.

? PROBABLY MYTH

Poppers burst your brain cells and you can hear it – that's why they're called poppers

If you read the opening paragraph to this chapter, you'll know how poppers got their colloquial name. But why did this myth come about? Do you know the current estimate for the number of brain cells in the human brain? It's around 100 billion. And when we're born, we have even more. We actually lose loads of brain cells in the first few years of life, and then again during adolescence, as our brains become streamlined and efficient. And once we're adults, brain cells still die every day.

It's certainly likely that some behaviours are more risky in terms of brain health, but as for poppers causing brain cells to 'pop', there is absolutely no evidence that this is the case, and even if it were, we wouldn't be able to hear them. We know that poppers cause a drop in blood pressure and a rush of blood to the head, and this can lead to a throbbing sensation in the ears. Maybe this has been mistaken for blood vessels popping by some people.

As for whether poppers are neurotoxic, we don't have very good evidence from humans. Some studies using mice or rats have suggested that poppers might impair learning and memory. However, it's worth pointing out here that rats in these studies were injected with various alkyl nitrites, which isn't the way that the liquids are consumed by people, so it's difficult to know how transferrable these findings are.

 MYTH

Poppers are psychoactive

In 2016, the UK government brought into effect what they called the Psychoactive Substances Bill – a piece of legislation that was intended to function as a blanket ban on all psychoactive substances (apart from the legal ones like caffeine, alcohol and tobacco), as a way of dealing with newly synthesised substances that were technically legal until they were made illegal by individual pieces of legislation. Initially, poppers were due to fall under this ban – and there was public outcry from many people, from politicians to academics.

The Advisory Council on the Misuse of Drugs wrote to the Home Office, and presented evidence that poppers are not, in fact, directly psychoactive. Their letter stated:

> The brain perceives a transient 'rush' or 'high' as an indirect effect caused by increased blood flow caused by the dilation of blood vessels in brain and periphery. The effects of 'poppers' on blood vessels in the brain should be considered to be 'peripheral' as these lie outside the 'blood-brain barrier' . . . The ACMD's consensus view is that a psychoactive substance has a direct action on the brain and that substances having peripheral effects, such as those caused by alkyl nitrites, do not directly stimulate or depress the central nervous system.*

In other words, they concluded that poppers were not psychoactive, and therefore shouldn't be included in the ban. And after consideration, then Home Secretary Theresa May accepted their recommendation, and poppers did not fall under the remit of the bill. However, more recently this correspondence between the ACMD and the Home Office has been legally challenged, with a court ruling that peripheral activation on the central

---

* Letter from Professor Les Iversen (Chair of ACMD) to Karen Bradley MP, Minister for preventing abuse, exploitation and crime, dated 16 March 2016.

nervous system would still be legally classed as a 'psychoactive effect'.

The court case was discussing nitrous oxide, rather than poppers, but even so it sets a legal precedent, and so no one is quite sure where poppers currently stand in terms of their legality. Having said all this, regardless of these legal wranglings, when poppers are sold they still have to be marketed as 'not for human consumption', as they are not a regulated product.

? UNCLEAR

Do alkyl nitrites have any medical uses?

Although initially developed as a medication, amyl nitrite fell out of favour as a treatment for angina in the early 1960s (as an aside, it was replaced by nitro-glycerine, probably better known as an explosive!). However, in some parts of the world, amyl nitrite is used as an antidote for cyanide poisoning. While it can treat cyanide poisoning, it is a risky method to do so compared to some other available treatments as it can create a toxic by-product, and is not as effective as some other methods. Having said that, it is relatively easy to administer.

Some researchers have investigated the potential for using amyl nitrite in cases of mass cyanide poisoning. A review of the animal and human literature on the use of amyl nitrite for cyanide poisoning concluded that the risks of side-effects are too high to warrant its use – side-effects such as hypotension (low blood pressure), syncope (fainting due to lack of blood flow to the brain), and the lack of accurate dosing due to administration from a cracked ampoule on a handkerchief. However, other researchers have suggested other potential methods of administration, such as via inhalers, to minimise this problem of poor dose control.

CHAPTER 20

Prescription Opioids

FENTANYL   MORPHINE   OXYCODONE

What is it? Many different pain-relieving medications, from buprenorphine to fentanyl, oxycodone or tramadol.

Type of drug: Depressant.

Popularity: Unfortunately growing in many countries.

How consumed: Via skin patch, swallowed, snorted or injected (into skin, muscle or blood).

Timescale: Varies depending on the particular substance.

Some effects: Pain relief, relaxation, nausea, slower and shallower breathing, weakened pulse.

THERE ARE NOT many days that go by at the moment where there isn't a news report discussing what is often referred to as the 'opioid crisis'. In the USA, but also Canada, Germany and other places around Europe, the consumption of opioids has been rising for some time, and so have opioid-related deaths. In the UK, opioid use is predominantly the use of heroin and morphine, but in other places around the world, opioid use can often refer to the use of prescription opioids.

Prescription opioids are medications prescribed for their pain-relieving properties. A number of medications fall under this title, including fentanyl, tramadol, buprenorphine, oxycodone, hydrocodone, codeine and morphine. They can be administered in a variety of different ways, which make them a useful and versatile pain medication. They can be given orally, as tablets or lozenges, they can be administered through the skin via a patch, and they can be administered via syringe, under the skin, into muscle, or directly into the bloodstream.

This chapter is a slightly different format to others in the book. If you're interested in the short- and long-term effects of opioids, have a read of the chapter about heroin, as they are broadly similar (although different opioids have slightly different profiles).

In this chapter, I'll explore a bit about why prescription opioids are appearing in a book that is not about prescribed medication.

Who uses prescription opioids?

Sometimes people who use opioids will begin to do so having been prescribed them by a doctor. This could be for a variety of illnesses, for recovery after surgery, chronic pain, or any number of reasons. Problematic use of prescription opioids can also be particularly common in professional sports people, either after treatment, or in a prophylactic way allowing them to play through injury, but without support to come off them. Sometimes opioids will be prescribed for severe pain, or managing pain after surgical procedures. Opioids are also extremely useful in end-of-life care – particularly for individuals with cancer pain.

Opioids of all kinds can induce pain relief, feelings of euphoria, and relaxation. They can also impact on breathing – slowing it down and making it shallower. They can cause constipation, which is why they're occasionally prescribed for people with diarrhoea. For some individuals, opioids can induce nausea, vomiting and dizziness, and reduce appetite.

There are a number of different opioids that are prescribed for many reasons and in a variety of circumstances. Some are synthetic, while others are semi-synthetic, having been derived from the opium poppy. Morphine and codeine are directly extracted from opium.

Perhaps the most well-known prescription opioid at present is fentanyl. This substance is synthetic – created in a lab – and similar to morphine, but around 50 to 100 times more potent. Fentanyl has had a lot of media attention because of its potency. This greatly increases risk of overdose, especially if the person consuming it is unaware that a powder or tablet contains fentanyl.

Overdose on opioids of all kinds is dangerous because they slow down a person's breathing rate. If breathing is slowed enough, a person can lose consciousness, and potentially die. Opioids are also dependence forming – after using them for a while, people require a higher dose to achieve the same pain-relieving effect, people can experience strong cravings for the substances, and people can experience unpleasant withdrawal symptoms if they stop taking them.

Cravings and withdrawal might be one reason why individuals who are initially prescribed opioids will sometimes continue taking them off-prescription, and tolerance may be a reason why individuals move from a lower-risk method of consumption like tablets to a higher-risk method such as injecting, where there are further dangers of infections, skin damage, and blood-borne diseases.

How effective are opioids as pain medication?

Opioids are extremely effective for the relief of acute – that is short-term – pain. Particularly pain that doesn't respond to what might be considered more standard pain medications, such as paracetamol, ibuprofen and aspirin. For all the risks we know about prescription opioids, are they actually any good at long-term pain relief?

The evidence is surprisingly thin on the ground. While they are proven to be an effective treatment for acute pain (such as pain following surgery), there's not that much evidence they are an effective treatment for longer-term pain, even before their dependence-forming risk is taken into account.

Public Health England have released guidance for clinicians when prescribing opioids, called 'Opioids Aware'. Their guidance states that while a small proportion of people might get a benefit from long-term use of opioids, it's very hard to identify who these people are, and benefit is often seen only when use is intermittent rather than continuous. They also state that use should be discontinued if a patient is still experiencing severe pain after taking opioids, even if there is no other treatment available.

In 2018, a clinical trial was published comparing the effectiveness of opioids including oxycodone, fentanyl and hydrocodone (known as the brand name Vicodin), in patients with back problems or knee or hip arthritis. A group of 234 mostly male participants were randomly prescribed either one of these opioids, or non-opioid pain medications ibuprofen or paracetamol, and followed up for a year. The participants rated their pain using questionnaires at the beginning of the trial, and at follow-up time-points.

The study found no difference in pain between the groups at the start (both rating their pain at around 5.5 on an 11-point scale). The non-opioid group reported an average lowering of two pain points at the end of the trial, and the opioid group a slightly smaller decrease. There was no evidence that opioids performed better as a long-term, pain-reduction treatment, and the authors of the study took their findings to mean that these risky medications should not be prescribed if they are no more effective than pain medications that don't have such a high risk for dependence or overdose.

If they're not that effective, why did opioids become so highly prescribed?

The rise of opioid popularity can be traced back to the USA in the 1990s. At this time, there was a huge outcry that pain was being under-treated. And while this outcry was happening, opioids were being advertised on TV as effective pain treatment. In the early 2000s, prescriptions for opioid pain medication in the USA boomed, but so did the use of the substances off-prescription or illicitly.

In 2012, opioids were the second most-common substance being used 'recreationally' (as opposed to being used as prescribed) in the USA, after cannabis. By 2014 it was estimated that over 10 million people in the USA were using opioids outside of prescription.

Why has problematic opioid use hit the USA harder than other places like the UK? It could be related to differences in the way healthcare is provided. In the USA, healthcare is privatised, and generally paid for via people's insurance. Alongside this, medications are advertised on TV, and doctors are offered incentives by pharmaceutical companies to prescribe certain medications.

The level of insurance that a person has might also impact on the type of treatment they get. For example, an individual with chronic back pain might benefit most greatly from an expensive, physical-therapy intervention, but have only a lower level of insurance, so may not be able to claim for anything other than pharmaceuticals that will mask the pain, rather than treat the underlying cause of the problem. However, given the rise in opioid prescribing elsewhere in the world such as Canada, and even the UK, where opioid prescription is rising, the explanation may not be this straightforward.

People who were initially prescribed them, particularly in the USA, and where prescriptions are expensive rather than subsidised by a national health service, might seek out cheaper illicit opioids when this becomes prohibitively expensive for them. There are additional risks from illicit use – heroin laced with fentanyl has been seen on the street, which people might knowingly or unknowingly buy and consume.

Where the substances are powders, they might be improperly or unevenly mixed together, making it very hard to predict the dosage accurately. And that is assuming the person knows the contents of the powder – there are huge risks from individuals consuming fentanyl when they believe it to be another, less-potent opioid, or another substance entirely.* In the UK, fentanyl is often found in base form, meaning it can be smoked or injected. In the USA, it is more common in salt form, which is only suitable for injection, a riskier method of consumption.

Why is it so hard to stop taking opioids?

Withdrawal from opioids can be extremely unpleasant – a heavy flu that can last a number of weeks, as well as anxiety, panic attacks and insomnia. And often the people who are using opioids

---

* There have been reports in the UK and the USA of fentanyl being sold as other substances, such as Xanax tablets.

are doing so for complex reasons such as chronic physical or emotional pain. The combination of these symptoms returning, plus the withdrawal symptoms, can be extremely hard to manage, particularly if they are trying to do so without support. Opioid withdrawal symptoms have been seen in the babies of women who used the substances while pregnant.

Some reports suggest that withdrawal symptoms are worse in people who use opioids recreationally rather than for a medicinal reason, but this might be due to taking higher doses, or a lack of support through the process of reducing the dose and stopping taking them.

Is there any way to make prescription opioids less harmful?

As detailed earlier, there are a number of different opioids, and each has its own unique profile, in terms of potency, onset and suchlike. As such, some opioids are less likely to lead to overdose, or dependence, than others. As well as this, efforts have been made to create less risky 'slow release' versions of some opioids.

For example, oxycodone is a fast-acting and long-lasting opioid – after consuming it in a tablet form, it will reach peak plasma concentration within thirty to sixty minutes and last for three to six hours. But a modified version has been created, where slow-release oxycodone is combined with naloxone, a substance that blocks the effect of an opioid directly at the receptors in the brain where opioids bind to take their effect. It's the same substance that can be used to reverse a heroin overdose, bringing people straight out into withdrawal, but possibly saving their lives.

The combination of oxycodone and naloxone might reduce the potential for dependence forming after use, and it also reduces the constipation that can be caused by opioid use. The peak plasma levels of oxycodone after taking the slow release version are at around three hours, rather than half an hour. This mixing of oxycodone and naloxone has a further benefit – when naloxone is taken orally, it doesn't stop the effect of oxycodone in the same way that it does when it's injected to prevent overdose, by blocking the receptor sites at synapses in the brain.

However, if an individual tries to grind up their oxycodone pills and inject them, the naloxone will be effective at blocking the oxycodone, meaning this isn't a viable way of consuming the substance. It is hoped that this will further reduce the risk of harm, by preventing injection as a consumption method.

Myths and misconceptions

You can overdose on fentanyl just by touching it

This is a really dangerous myth. It began with media reports of police officers in the USA reportedly falling unconscious after touching powder believed to be fentanyl. A police officer was said to have collapsed after brushing a small amount of fentanyl powder off his uniform. More scary still, despite being administered with naloxone he could not be revived immediately (though in all instances where this has occurred, the officers have made full recoveries).

It is vanishingly unlikely that these officers collapsed due to touching fentanyl. While it is possible for fentanyl to be absorbed through the skin, an individual would need to be exposed to a large amount of the substance, for a prolonged period of time. There is a risk if fentanyl powder becomes airborne and it is breathed in, but again the amount of fentanyl in the air is unlikely to be encountered by police officers at a crime scene.

The American College of Medical Toxicology has published a position statement after these reports started appearing. They point out that the symptoms reported by these police officers were not that consistent with an opioid overdose. Overdose symptoms might include slowed or shallow breathing, rather than dizziness or anxiety, which were examples of the symptoms reported by police officers.

Some have suggested the officers may have been having severe panic attacks rather than experiencing opioid overdose. And who could blame them – if you'd heard that this substance could kill you simply by touching it, then experiencing extreme fear at doing so is a natural response.

This myth is potentially a danger to emergency responders, but it's also a danger to individuals who might be at risk of overdose from fentanyl – if emergency responders believe they need to take extreme precautions before entering an area where fentanyl might be present, this could delay their ability to provide life-saving interventions like naloxone.

✗ **MYTH**

What can be done about the opioid crisis, and rising deaths from opioids?

While the President of the USA has declared the rising death toll from opioids as a public-health emergency in the USA, and there are many lawsuits being filed against drug companies who market these substances, what is being done to prevent deaths in the USA, and elsewhere?

There are a number of different levels at which this problem can be tackled. In the UK, for example, some police forces have been provided with naloxone, which can be used to bring a person who is overdosing out of intoxication and hopefully save their life. In Canada, as we have heard earlier, the government are encouraging organisations to set up drug consumption rooms, where individuals can go and take substances in a cleaner, safer environment than having to do so clandestinely on the street. These rooms can also test substances for the presence of adulterants, test individuals for blood-borne diseases, and provide education and social support.

There is currently a call for such provision to be provided in Scotland, where deaths from opioids are extremely high, on a par with the USA percentage-wise. Unfortunately, across the UK, drug-treatment services have been cut dramatically over recent years, meaning people who are vulnerable and at risk are in all likelihood finding it much harder to get support.

At the other end of the scale, we need better understanding of why opioids are being (over-)prescribed in such volume in certain countries around the world, and whether there are other options for dealing with chronic pain that are more effective, and less risky.

CHAPTER 21

Psilocybin:
Magic Mushrooms

PSILOCYBIN

What is it? Active compound in magic mushrooms (yes, actual mushrooms).

Type of drug: Psychedelic.

Popularity: Broadly similar to other psychedelics.

How consumed: Eaten, or drunk in a tea.

Timescale: Onset within an hour, can last for several hours.

Some effects: Perceptual alterations, time distortion, vivid colours and shapes, mood alterations, can cause stomach pain.

WHEN PEOPLE REFER to magic mushrooms, for the most part they are talking about mushrooms that contain a psychedelic substance called psilocybin. It is not one particular species of fungus that contains the substance, in fact estimates suggest about 180 different species of mushroom contain psilocybin.

Despite one being synthetic and one being naturally occurring, the story of psilocybin and the story of LSD go at least partly hand in hand. Albert Hofmann, the chemist who discovered LSD, was also the first person to isolate psilocybin from a mushroom. Timothy Leary's Harvard research, and the subsequent psychedelic counterculture revolution that in part it inspired, utilised both LSD and mushrooms. And this perhaps isn't surprising, as psilocybin and LSD molecules are very similar – both bearing a strong resemblance to serotonin, a neurotransmitter found in our brains involved in regulating mood, appetite and sleep, among other things.

While LSD is more popular among older people, mushrooms are the most commonly used psychedelic among young people (those aged thirty-four and under) – certainly in the USA. Mushrooms might be appealing because they are natural rather than synthetic (although as we've seen in other chapters, being natural doesn't necessarily mean being safer).

It may also be because they grow naturally in many parts of the world, including around the UK, which means if people know what they are looking for, they can forage for mushrooms themselves, or even grow their own, rather than buying them (although this is risky as there are also many poisonous mushrooms that look similar). And not too long ago, it wasn't illegal to buy or sell mushrooms in certain conditions in Britain.

As a teenager, I used to get the train up to London on a Sunday to roam around Camden Town trying on vintage coats and wearing too much eyeliner. I can vividly remember the shops selling mushrooms that lined the high street. Perhaps this combination of easy access and a perceived lower risk makes psilocybin appealing, particularly to young people. Although the difference in prevalence between LSD and mushrooms is small.

A 2016 prevalence survey in the USA called 'Monitoring the Future' put past-year LSD use at around 3 per cent in young adults, while non-LSD hallucinogen use was slightly higher, at around 3.5 per cent. A 2015 survey also in the USA, the National Survey on Drug Use and Health, found the proportion of adults of all ages who said they had ever tried LSD was slightly higher than for mushrooms, at around 9.5 per cent compared to about 8.5 per cent. A similar survey in the UK put past-year prevalence of LSD at less than 1 per cent in young adults, while mushroom use was slightly higher at around 1 per cent.

What are the short-term effects?

It's not unusual to consume mushrooms in a tea – you can eat dried or even fresh mushrooms by themselves, but they don't taste particularly nice, so people tend to try and hide them in other food to mask the taste or drink them quickly.

Intoxication intensity and duration will depend upon the dose of mushrooms that you consume, but intoxication usually begins at around thirty minutes after consumption, and a trip can last for four to six hours. The intoxication experience is broadly similar to that of LSD. People report experiencing perceptual distortion, often fractal-type imagery, a shifting of patterns when they are observed, or halos around objects.

Researchers in the field inform me that true hallucinations are not common – people experience perceptual alterations or pseudo-hallucinations, but remain aware that what they are seeing or experiencing is not actually happening. Some experience synaesthesia-like experiences, where senses that don't usually overlap start to do so – people can report sounds becoming 'colourful', or being able to smell words, for example. People can get extremely giggly while on mushrooms, but it can have other effects on emotion as well, and some people might get scared or anxious.

There are many different species of mushroom that contain psilocybin, though most are small and brown or tan, and found in the genuses *Psilocybe*, *Panaeolus* and *Copelandia*, and the potency of different species can vary. A study conducted in 1982 tested twenty different species of mushroom that grow in the Pacific Northwest and found psilocybin present in seven of them. Even within the same species, the amount of psilocybin varied by more than a factor of seven between different collection events. The researchers found that levels of psilocybin and psilocin varied from between 0.1 per cent to nearly 2 per cent by dry weight of mushroom. Even when growing mushrooms themselves, they found that levels of psilocybin varied from one fruiting to the next.

Because of the consumption of the plant matter of the mushroom, along with the psilocybin it contains, people can sometimes experience stomach cramps after eating them. Mushrooms can also give a person diarrhoea, or make them dizzy or nauseous. This doesn't occur as often or intensely when isolated or synthesised psilocybin is injected or consumed (more on that later), although dizziness and nausea can still sometimes occur.

What are the longer-term effects?

Longer term, there is little evidence that use of magic mushrooms can lead to addiction, similarly to other psychedelics. Some people report headaches after use, which might occur in the twenty-four hours after taking mushrooms. Much like other psychedelics, psilocybin can be particularly risky to consume for people with a predisposition to poor mental health, in particular people with a family history of psychosis or schizophrenia, as it is possible psychedelics can trigger latent psychotic symptoms or disorders.

Myths and misconceptions

Mushrooms are responsible for human cognition taking a great leap forward

This is a really interesting one – it's also sometimes called the Stoned Ape hypothesis. It was conceived by Terence McKenna, an author and lecturer, sometimes referred to as 'the Timothy Leary of the 90s'. He posited that magic mushrooms might be responsible for the leap in cognition and social organisation between *homo erectus* and *homo sapiens*, basically that psilocybin led to enlightenment and human evolution.

He believed that ingestion of a small amount of mushroom would improve vision and therefore hunting ability, a larger amount would encourage copulation and therefore lead to more offspring, and that higher doses still would act to dissolve hierarchy, encourage group sex, and stimulate the language areas in the brain, encouraging the creation of art and music, and catalysing the beginning of language in humans.

While at face value there's something quite appealing to this – mushrooms causing consciousness expansion – his arguments don't really stand up to scrutiny on closer inspection. It is perfectly possible that psilocybin-containing mushrooms could have been present in areas where *homo erectus* lived, but McKenna's theory doesn't really reference the swathes of evidence from paleoanthropology that have investigated this period in human evolution.

Some of his hypotheses, for example around the impact of small doses of psilocybin on vision, don't seem to be supported by research that has looked at the impact of the substance on human visual ability. Similarly, there's little evidence that use of mushrooms increases sex drive and would lead to more offspring. Also, in early cultures where use of psychedelics has been recorded, for example among Amazonian tribes, the societal dynamics he predicts in his theory are not seen.

McKenna believed lots of interesting things about psilocybin – another particularly wild theory he espoused was that mushrooms are actually an advanced species of high intelligence from another planet, whose spores had drifted to earth from elsewhere and were trying to communicate with humans via the psychedelic experience. He also speculated that a psychedelic trip could be a form of trans-dimensional travel, or a 'doorway into the Gaian mind' – a way to speak directly to the planet. All these theories are, of course, very hard to prove – or disprove.

? UNCLEAR

Mushrooms are just 'natural LSD'

While psilocybin and LSD are chemically very similar, they are not identical, and certainly the intoxication experience is reportedly slightly different between the two substances, although as discussed in the LSD chapter, how much of this is due to expectation effect is hard to tease out. A related myth, that LSD is extracted from magic mushrooms, is similarly false. Although LSD was in fact derived from ergot, which is also a fungus.* As I have described earlier, LSD was derived by Albert Hofmann before psilocybin had been isolated from mushrooms, which was also done by Dr Hofmann more than a decade after he discovered LSD.

There are also known pharmacological differences in the action of LSD and psilocybin, that might further explain some of the differences in subjective effects of the two. For example, while both substances have an effect on serotonin receptor action, there is evidence that LSD has an impact on certain

---

* In this regard, LSD is semi-synthetic, since it was synthesised from a naturally occurring compound.

dopamine receptors known as D2 receptors, that psilocybin does not have.

 MYTH

All psychedelic mushrooms bruise blue

Do mushrooms bruise? Well, yes, if you squeeze the stem or the cap, this can cause some discolouration – a bruise. Some people claim this is a good way to identify whether a mushroom is psychedelic or not, but actually it is not accurate enough to do so reliably, not without other information as well. Some mushrooms containing psilocybin will not bruise blue, and some mushrooms that don't contain it will.

Mycologists might use bruising colour in the final stages of identification of a certain species of mushroom, as it can help to differentiate between two otherwise very similar-looking species, but if you don't have this other knowledge, bruising colour will probably not help you, and could put you at risk of ingesting a toxic mushroom.

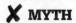 **MYTH**

Does psilocybin have any medical uses?

In recent years, there has been a growing body of research conducted into the potential therapeutic effects of psilocybin. So far, these studies have been on a very small scale, often with less than twenty individuals sampled. Researchers in the UK gave fifteen healthy individuals, who were experienced with using psychedelics, either psilocybin or placebo intravenously, on two separate occasions.

While they were intoxicated, they were put in an MRI scanner, which is essentially a giant electromagnet that uses pulses of radio waves to align the spin of protons in the water molecules in whatever bit of the body is in the scanner (in this case the head). Transmitters within the scanner can then pick up information about this spin alignment. Differences in the spin can indicate what type of tissue or cell is present in certain areas of the brain. As well as that, it can give information about function or activity in the brain, inferred by the oxygenation level of blood in different brain areas, which affects the spin alignment.

Researchers used the scanner to measure blood flow during placebo, and during psilocybin intoxication, and compared the findings. They were surprised to see that blood flow was decreased while the participants were on psilocybin. This decrease was particularly striking in known 'hub' areas of the brain – areas that showed especially high levels of blood flow in the placebo condition.

To investigate their findings further these researchers, along with colleagues in Italy, used the functional-imaging scans to derive brain-connectivity data. The picture they generated from the data was quite striking. Whilst on placebo, connections in the brain were mostly streamlined and within functional areas – vision areas of the brain were connected to other vision areas, and so on. The picture of the psilocybin-intoxicated brain by contrast showed connections across the gamut of brain regions.

The image they present in their paper looks like a child's spirograph gone wrong – disparate points are joined up where previously they were unconnected. There were no extra connections, the total number was the same, but the way these connections crossed between brain regions was completely different. The researchers found these connections were not random, and seemed to be stable while the individual was intoxicated, returning to the more expected pattern afterwards.

What might these findings mean? The authors interpret them

as evidence of a dampening of the 'usual' brain connections during psilocybin, allowing less-used connections to occur. They also highlight the relevance of their findings to the potential for psilocybin to be used as a treatment for depression, pointing out that certain brain areas that are overactive in people with depression – such as the prefrontal cortex – were the same areas showing lower blood flow during psilocybin intoxication.

Does psilocybin have any therapeutic effect? So far, the evidence is mainly based upon small studies, mostly without placebo controls, and with very small sample sizes. But research is being conducted to investigate the impact of psilocybin on a number of conditions that people anecdotally report being improved by mushrooms. These include cluster headaches and depression. As well as that, trials are underway in the USA and in the UK investigating the potential for the use of psilocybin as a treatment for addiction to various substances, particularly alcohol and tobacco, and even as a treatment for helping patients with a terminal illness come to terms with their diagnosis and its implications.

What does treatment with psilocybin look like? Firstly, it's important to stress that a person isn't merely given the drug and then sent on their way. The substance is administered as part of an intensive therapy, by trained psychologists or psychotherapists, with thorough preparation before psilocybin is administered, and dedicated integration sessions to process the experience afterwards.

There are a couple of different ways that this can happen. In some cases, talking therapy occurs while a person is intoxicated, usually under the influence of a low dose of psilocybin. In others, the psilocybin experience plays out without discussion, and then the participant will be invited to talk about it afterwards. Dr Albert Garcia-Romeu, one of the researchers who ran some of these studies at Johns Hopkins University in Baltimore, described it as like watching a film. You wouldn't talk all the way through a movie, you wait until it's finished.

He told me about the setup for running these studies. A lot of thought goes into the room in which a person will have their psilocybin session. Set and setting, as we've discussed throughout this book, is extremely important in influencing the type of intoxication experience. Participants lie on a bed or a sofa in a softly lit room. They will wear an eye mask, and headphones with a carefully curated soundtrack. Someone will be with them throughout their intoxication experience, on-hand in case they experience any distress. And they will already know and trust this person – in fact the participant will typically have had a month of therapy before any drug is administered to them.

This will be something like cognitive behavioural therapy or motivational enhancement therapy, and will be tailored to whatever the trial is investigating, for example the therapy might focus on smoking behaviour, barriers to quitting and motivations to quit, as well as a life review, to understand where the participant is in their life, and how smoking has played a role in their life. Sometimes a trial protocol will administer psilocybin only once, sometimes up to three times, with aftercare between each psilocybin session.

So far, these trials are finding tantalising hints that psilocybin could have some therapeutic potential, in certain circumstances, for some people, for a variety of conditions. Having said that, we are a long way off our doctors prescribing us mushrooms. These studies are done in small numbers of individuals who opt in to take part, although participant numbers are increasing in more recent studies.

It is also notoriously difficult to blind studies using psychedelics – even if a participant doesn't know they've been given psilocybin, as soon as the substance takes effect it will in all likelihood become apparent to both participant and experimenter. Recent study designs are trying to get around this by giving what are known as active placebos – substances that have an effect in some ways similar to that of the substance being researched.

In the case of psilocybin, some studies have used psychoactive substances such as niacin, ephedrine, methylphenidate or even lower doses of a psychedelic. Even so, research has found that trained session moderators are able to ascertain correctly the condition of a participant in such studies somewhere between 77 to 95 per cent of the time.

What don't we know?

There are other types of hallucinogenic mushroom, which contain different substances to psilocybin. Probably the most well-known is fly agaric. If you picture a toadstool, you're probably picturing fly agaric – a white stem, and a red cap with white spots. There's far less research around fly agaric than there is around psilocybin, but the active chemicals thought to give the psychedelic effect are muscimol and ibotenic acid.

Anecdotal reports suggest that the intoxication effect of fly agaric is broadly similar to psilocybin-containing mushrooms, but slightly less pleasant, and potentially with more unwanted side-effects, including sweating and stomach cramps. It is also possible to experience severe health problems after eating fly agaric, some estimates suggest consuming around fifteen caps could be a lethal dose of the mushroom.

Focus on: Stimulants

Sometimes referred to as uppers, stimulants are, as the name suggests, substances that increase certain facets of body and mind. Stimulants can be consumed in many different ways, which will impact the intensity and duration of intoxication, from chewing coca or khat leaves, to drinking coffee, swallowing amphetamine tablets, snorting cocaine powder, smoking cigarettes or in extreme cases injecting crack cocaine.

Which drugs are stimulants?

Stimulants make up a large number of the drugs covered in this book, from the commonly used caffeine, the decreasingly popular but still legal nicotine, to illicit drugs like cocaine and amphetamine. Other substances might not be considered pure stimulants, but still have some of the key properties of a stimulant.

For example, MDMA is sometimes called an empathogen or an entactogen due to its impact on emotion and feelings of connectedness to others, but it would also be considered a stimulant due to its impact on energy, alertness and physiology. Khat and related synthetic cathinones are also stimulants.

What effects do stimulants have?

Stimulants increase blood pressure, heart rate and body temperature. They might make a person feel more alert and awake, and can even induce feelings of euphoria – but can also make people feel paranoid, anxious or irritable. These substances might make a person feel more confident, induce feelings of wellbeing, motivation or focus. They might make a person feel more social, they might even make a person feel more horny, or increase their sex drive.

Stimulants are appetite suppressants, so might make a person feel less hungry. They can also often cause dry mouth. As might be expected of a substance that increases feelings of alertness, stimulants can make it harder to sleep, and can induce feelings of restlessness.

At higher doses, stimulants can put pressure on the heart, and the risk of heart attack or stroke is possible for a number of the drugs in this category. There is also a potential risk of hyperthermia – the body overheating.

Stimulants have the potential to lead to dependence – again this is influenced by how the substance is consumed, with methods of consumption that lead to faster absorption into the bloodstream increasing the risk. Stimulants are risky substances to take if a person suffers from heart problems or blood pressure problems, as increased strain is put on the circulatory system.

Interactions

It is dangerous to mix stimulants with other stimulants. The more substances you take that ramp up the body's heart rate, blood pressure and temperature, the more pressure you're putting on those systems, and the higher the risk. But it can also be risky to mix stimulants with depressants like alcohol or GHB. Doing so can mean each substance masks the effect of the other, which might lead a person to think they are less intoxicated than they are and cause them problems, because they feel more sober than they really are. It might also result in an individual taking more of each substance than they otherwise would, putting extra strain on their body, including on the liver that will need to metabolise the substances.

CHAPTER 22

Salvia

SALVINORIN A

What is it? Found in the leaves of a type of mint plant, in the sage family.

Type of drug: A bit dissociative, a bit psychedelic – hard to pin down.

Popularity: Unclear – it's not a substance commonly asked about in surveys.

How consumed: Fresh leaves can be chewed, or dried leaves can be smoked or made into tea.

Timescale: Depends on method of consumption, but short compared to other psychedelics, intoxication is usually over within an hour.

Some effects: Giggly, depersonalisation, can impact on ability to remember you have taken a substance, inability to remember who you are.

SALVIA DIVINORUM IS the species name for a plant – a type of mint from the sage family. There are many non-psychoactive types of salvia too, in fact you can find pretty flowering salvia plants in most garden centres up and down the country. The 'divinorum' in the name is thought to be in reference to traditional use of the plant in medicinal divination – as you may know if you're a Harry Potter fan, divination is the act of foreseeing or prophesying. Medical divination means using oracles and prophecy to treat medical complaints or illnesses.

Salvia plants have large green leaves and purply-white flowers. The plant grows native to southern Mexico (the Oaxaca region), but can be cultivated in many parts of the world. It has been used by Mazatec people there for hundreds of years – within rituals and spiritual experiences, as a herbal remedy for various health complaints, and in the practice of medical divination, mentioned above. Some researchers believe it to be a hybrid plant – the result of selective pollination over many years.

A compound found within the leaves, called Salvinorin A, has been the most widely researched, and is thought to be involved in the psychoactive effects of the plant. Salvia has been described by people who have used it as having both a dissociative and a psychedelic intoxication effect. It is an unusual psychoactive drug compared to what we might think of as 'classic' psychedelics such as LSD, psilocybin or DMT.

At a molecular level, the structure of salvia is very different from these substances, all of which are very similar. It's also quite different in structure to other drugs that have a dissociative effect, like ketamine. Although recently, there have been some suggestions that both salvia and ketamine produce their effects by interacting at locations in the brain called k-opioid receptors, which are part of the opioid system. It's not really clear yet to researchers why this action would lead to the effects that are experienced by people who use salvia, though.

In fact, there's very little research into salvia. I'm aware I say that for a lot of drugs in this book, but this is particularly the case for salvia. There's not even any research into how many people use salvia in the UK. There's a little more information in the USA – I spoke to Dr Joseph Palamar, a drug researcher at New York University, on Twitter and he told me that surveys in the US suggest that around 3.4 per cent of eighteen- to twenty-five-year-olds there had ever tried salvia, while roughly 6.3 per cent of twenty-six- to thirty-four-year-olds ever had. The number of people who had used it in the past year was much lower, less than 0.5 per cent.

How salvia causes the experiences it does is poorly understood and we know relatively little about who uses salvia recreationally, how often, and why. So when you're reading the rest of this chapter, do bear that in mind, because although I'll talk about things like prevalence of use, potential reasons for using, and some of the short- and long-term effects of the substance, this is based on only small amounts of evidence. This doesn't mean it's wrong, but it means there might be a lot of uncertainty around any estimates made.

Why might salvia appeal? Compared to other psychedelics (perhaps with the exception of DMT), salvia gives a much shorter intoxication experience. This might make it more appealing to some. It's also more intense, certainly at higher doses, than LSD or mushrooms. Until the Psychoactive Substances Bill was brought into the UK in 2016, salvia was legal, which might have given some people the impression that it was a (relatively) safe substance. But that is not necessarily the case.

What are the short-term effects?

Salvia can be consumed in a few ways. Fresh leaves can be held in the mouth and chewed so the Salvinorin A is released into the mouth and absorbed into the bloodstream from there. Dried salvia leaves can be smoked or made into a drink by mixing with water. Dried leaves lose some of their potency, so these are often sold in a concentrated way, where the leaves have been sprayed or coated with extra Salvinorin A, so sometimes dried salvia can be sold at various different concentrations. The preparations can be flavoured with fruit extracts to make them more palatable, and concentrated solutions or tinctures of salvia are also available in some places.

Using substances that have had psychoactive compounds sprayed on them can be really risky. Given the illicit nature of these substances in the UK,* there's obviously no quality control here. What a person purchases may bear little or no relation to what they wanted. Not only that, but often the method of spraying can lead to some dried leaves being extremely strong, while others will have no added Salvinorin A at all. There's a real lack of consistency possible. This can lead to accidentally consuming far more than intended, which can have pretty unpleasant consequences, as we'll get onto below.

As with all substances, the method of consumption will impact on the time to onset, and the length of intoxication. If smoking salvia, the onset of intoxication will occur within seconds. It will peak at around five to ten minutes, and be over within half an hour. Chewing leaves is slowed, with intoxication onset at around fifteen minutes, a peak of intoxication at around half an hour, and intoxication ending at around an hour.

Much like other psychedelics, salvia's effects are somewhat dose dependent. At low levels, people report feeling 'odd'. Some will get giggly, some will feel strange. This isn't a million miles away from low doses of psychedelics, like mushrooms, or

---

* Salvia was actually not illegal in the UK before the Psychoactive Substances Bill was passed in 2016. Its legal status is varied across the world, being controlled in the USA, Japan, Australia, Italy, Spain, Canada, and a number of other countries, but legal in other places such as France, Austria and Thailand. Of course, even where it is legal, it is not regulated and therefore these risks will still apply.

dissociative substances, like ketamine. At higher doses, experiences become more psychedelic, and there are more reports of depersonalisation or derealisation experiences.*

Some hallucinatory experiences are similar to those from other psychedelics, but some are quite different, or more extreme. In particular, people who use salvia report more severe time-perception alterations from salvia compared to other psychedelics. Salvia intoxication seems to be a full-body experience: people report feeling as if they are falling, or they are being pulled or dragged around.

At very high doses, effects can get even more extreme. It is not uncommon for people to lose the ability to remember that they have taken a drug, and some people cannot remember who they are. Some people report encounters with other beings, or complete emergence in an alternate reality during intoxication. Spiritual experiences are also sometimes reported.

A survey conducted in the UK in 2010 asked people who use salvia why they took it. Some reported using it for self-exploration or for what they referred to as 'personal psychotherapy'.† Although some people do report pleasurable experiences from salvia intoxication such as calmness and relaxation, improved mood, or an intensification of sensual experiences, it is common for a salvia trip not to be pleasurable.

The survey also found people reporting audio (but not visual) hallucinations, feeling socially withdrawn, mental confusion, amnesia and anxiety after taking salvia. They also reported psychomotor dysfunction – it would be terribly dangerous to drive while

---

* Depersonalisation is the feeling of losing the sense of who you are. Derealisation is losing the sense of what is real around you, or losing trust in being able to tell.

† It goes without saying (but I'm saying it anyway) that a psychedelic or dissociative trip is in no way equivalent to psychotherapy from a qualified therapist, and really shouldn't be seen in that way.

under the influence of salvia, and it may also be risky to consume it in a public place.

Salvia intoxication can induce hallucinations or perceptual changes that might encourage the person experiencing them to want to get up and move around while intoxicated. So thinking about where, when, and with whom you take salvia is extremely important if you are considering using it. Being in a location where you can't hurt yourself is vital, and (this is true for all psychedelics, but particularly for salvia) it is strongly advisable to have a sitter with you if you choose to take it, who can look after you until the intoxication experience is over, even if you are used to taking psychedelics.

Something that people who use salvia report, which is different from other psychedelics, is the feeling that the trip is something happening to them, rather than something that they are involved with or part of. Less pleasant symptoms of salvia intoxication include confusion and disorientation (not very surprising considering the previous paragraphs), fear, dizziness and an increased heart rate. Some people have said they felt like they were dying, or like they were going permanently mad while intoxicated on salvia.

However, for all these unpleasant intoxication effects, there is little evidence to suggest that salvia is toxic to the human body, or physically harmful. If a person 'overdoses' on salvia, they will have a more extreme or intense trip. At the moment, there has not been any research that has investigated the long-term impact of overdosing on salvia, but there have not been reports of people experiencing physical harm from doing so, other than those who injure themselves while intoxicated.

What are the longer-term effects?

The longer-term effects of salvia are mainly based on anecdote. Lung irritation is one such effect, which is perhaps not surprising given some people will be smoking salvia, and therefore inhaling carcinogens from burning plant matter (even though salvia is not mixed with tobacco). There is, as far as I can see, only one documented case of a person developing psychosis after using salvia, which means it's impossible to draw too many conclusions from that.

More common, although still only anecdotal, are reports of persisting unpleasant effects in the days or possibly weeks following use of salvia. These can include feelings of derealisation persisting for a couple of days, or possibly flashbacks, but as yet there's no good-quality scientific evidence as to the rates at which these are occurring, or the severity. Salvia can also make individuals feel 'foggy' or experience headaches in the hours or days following intoxication. Like other psychedelics, salvia does not seem to be habit-forming.

Perhaps surprisingly, although people often have trips they would not class as pleasant, few individuals have reported regretting using salvia, when asked. Salvia is not a drug that people who use it tend to take very frequently, possibly because it is an unusual intoxication experience, and not uniformly pleasant.

However, it is a substance that people seem keen to document – there is a trend for posting videos of salvia intoxication to YouTube. Probably the most (in)famous of these features none other than Miley Cyrus. Whether she's actually taking salvia or not is up for debate, but the media who shared the video reported that she was.

Myths and misconceptions

Salvia is like cannabis

Because salvia is often purchased as either fresh or dried leaves, and is commonly smoked, some can erroneously believe that the effects will therefore be similar to cannabis, or perhaps similar to synthetic cannabinoids. As can be seen clearly from the descriptions above, this is very much not the case. Salvia has also been sold under the name 'herbal ecstasy' or sometimes 'horse killer', but the intoxication experience is not very similar to MDMA, so this is not a particularly accurate description either.

 MYTH

Does salvia have any medical uses?

At the moment, there's no good-quality evidence that salvia has any medical benefits. Among the population in the region of Mexico where salvia grows naturally, it has for many years been used as a herbal remedy to treat conditions such as migraine, rheumatoid arthritis and diarrhoea. More recently, researchers in the USA have begun to investigate the potential for salvia as a treatment for other addictions, due to its suspected action on k-opioid receptors.

As yet this is very early days, and there has been nothing conclusive found, but it's interesting. However, would people really be keen to take a substance that has such an intense psychedelic experience? It's hard to say – ketamine is perhaps the most comparable substance to salvia in terms of this experience, and it is also being researched for similar purposes, so perhaps salvia would also be viable.

CHAPTER 23

Synthetic Cannabinoids: Spice, K2 and others

What are they? Synthetic substances initially designed as research chemicals, looking to mimic the effects of compounds found in herbal cannabis.

Type of drug: Cannabinoid (related to but not identical to those found in herbal cannabis, or the endocannabinoids that we produce ourselves).

Popularity: Particularly used among the homeless and prison populations.

How consumed: Smoked, vaped or made into tea.

Some effects: Elevated mood, relaxation, perceptual alterations, increased appetite, aggression, vomiting, dangerously high body temperature, seizures.

PERHAPS YOU'VE HEARD of Spice? No, not the mysterious drug from David Lynch's sci-fi movie *Dune* (worth checking out if you've not seen it, if you're a fan of incomprehensibility and Sting in little blue pants), but slang for synthetic cannabinoids – a group of substances that have been growing in popularity in the UK and elsewhere since they first started appearing for sale in the early 2000s.

Initially developed as research chemicals, they were part of a group of chemicals that grew up on the fringes of legality, certainly in the UK. Until 2016's Psychoactive Substances Bill, drugs were classed as controlled on a case-by-case basis. A small tweak to a compound and it would no longer be covered by the ban, meaning substances could be technically marketed as a 'legal high'. A synthetic cannabinoid would appear, be banned, was tweaked, and reappeared as a slightly different substance, no longer controlled. And they made a whole lot of newspaper headlines along the way, as we'll see.

What are they?

Sometimes referred to as new or novel psychoactive substances (NPS), synthetic cannabinoids is a collective term that refers to a wide range of different substances that affect cannabinoid receptors in the brain (and sometimes the cannabinoid receptors outside the central nervous system, too). Whilst they share some similarities to herbal cannabis and the more extensively researched compounds in the cannabis plant (such as THC), the effects of many synthetic cannabinoids on the body and brain can be more extreme and they shouldn't just be considered lab-made versions of herbal cannabis, or 'synthetic cannabis'.

Synthetic cannabinoids are sold under many names, but 'spice' is one of the most widely known, and is often used as an umbrella term for all types of synthetic cannabinoids in the UK. However, there is regional and national variation in the terms used to describe synthetic cannabinoids – of which some estimate there are over 400 types available, and other names the substances are sold under have included K2, Joker, Black Mamba, Cowboy Kush and Kronic.

Synthetic cannabinoids are often sold sprayed onto a dried plant material, resembling tobacco leaf. This is then smoked or made into a tea. It is also possible to vape synthetic cannabinoids dissolved in an appropriate fluid. In the USA, some vaping liquids sold as cannabidiol (CBD – a compound found in cannabis) have been found to contain synthetic cannabinoids.

Synthetic cannabinoids were initially appealing because they were perceived as a cheap and legal alternative to cannabis. As they were often sold in shops or online, they were generally easier to get hold of than cannabis, and the legal status may have meant that some people thought they were safer.

In the USA, they gained popularity as they were not detectable in drug-screening tests, meaning people who were regularly subject to such tests – university and school athletes, members of the armed forces, individuals on parole, healthcare professionals and shift workers – might have been tempted to use these over herbal cannabis, which was easily detected in screens, up to several weeks after last use.

Similarly to the USA, synthetic cannabinoids became popular in prisons in the UK because they didn't have the familiar odour of cannabis, weren't detected by drug screens or sniffer dogs, and were easy to smuggle in, either inside the body or impregnated onto paper or fabrics.

What are the short-term effects?

If a person smokes or otherwise consumes a synthetic cannabinoid, they may experience intoxication that feels similar-ish to that from herbal cannabis. For example, they might have an elevated mood and feelings of relaxation. They might also experience perceptual alterations. It is likely to increase a person's appetite, and can make people feel sleepy, although it has also been associated with increasing aggressiveness and violence.

Some people may report psychotic-like symptoms including confusion, paranoia, anxiety and hallucinations. So far, so like cannabis, but people who use synthetic cannabinoids report psychotic-like experiences much more frequently, and more severely, than those who use herbal cannabis. Synthetic cannabinoids can induce nausea and vomiting – there are even case reports of individuals experiencing hyperemesis after synthetic cannabinoid use. Hyperemesis is a condition characterised by severe and prolonged vomiting, often requiring hospitalisation as it can lead to dehydration. Synthetic cannabinoids also increase heart rate, and have been linked to risk of seizures.

Use of these substances has been responsible for mass poisonings and many trips to emergency rooms across the USA and Europe, often with symptoms that are not seen after herbal cannabis. For example, there is some evidence that synthetic cannabinoids at high doses can cause an individual's body temperature to rise very rapidly, which can put the person at risk of coma and of damage to their vital organs. Doctors have reported cases of patients with kidney damage, heart attacks, or stroke.

Synthetic cannabinoid intoxication has also been implicated in cases of violence, leading some to believe that it causes the behaviour (although this is hard to be certain about, for reasons I'll go into later).

What are the longer-term effects?

We know little about the longer-term impact of regular synthetic cannabinoid use. Synthetic cannabinoids first became popular recreationally in the early 2000s, but the research community took a while to catch up with what people were using, and they only began to be identified by drug sample tests several years later. This is often the case, particularly with new substances, where molecular tweaks mean new variants emerge all the time – it can be hard for research to keep up and keep on top of understanding the effects of them.

If people are smoking synthetic cannabinoids sprayed onto dried plant material, then it is likely that some similar risks to that of smoking tobacco may be expected due to the nature of inhaling burning plant matter (and this might lead to other harms too, detailed later).

There are a growing number of case studies indicating that synthetic cannabinoids can trigger psychosis above and beyond the transient symptoms seen during intoxication. These case reports are also seen after use of herbal cannabis, although many people researching these substances believe that the risk of psychosis is far greater for synthetic cannabinoids than for herbal cannabis.

A recent paper published by researchers across Europe recruited 367 individuals who used herbal cannabis or synthetic canna-binoids, and gave them a battery of questionnaires. The 238 synthetic cannabinoid users were different from the 129 herbal cannabis users in a number of ways. Synthetic cannabinoid use was associated with higher scores on all measures of general or specific psychopathology the researchers measured, including insomnia, mania, and a global measure investigating symptoms of a number of different mental health problems including depression, anxiety, psychosis symptoms and paranoia.

It is worth pointing out that around 80 per cent of the synthetic cannabinoid group were also using herbal cannabis, and were more likely than the herbal cannabis group to be using a number of other illicit substances. Even so, in this sample, synthetic cannabinoid use was predictive of up to over five times greater risk of poor mental health. This study cannot tell us about causality – it's impossible to tell whether people with poorer mental health are drawn to use synthetic cannabinoids, or whether the synthetic cannabinoids might be increasing the risk – but it's potentially worrying, nonetheless.

People working in emergency departments have published articles detailing how challenging it can be to diagnose synthetic cannabinoid intoxication. Firstly, this is because synthetic cannabinoids will often not be picked up by a typical drug-screening procedure. Also, physicians have noted that symptoms of synthetic cannabinoid intoxication can look very similar to that of serotonin syndrome – a disorder that can occur after consumption of certain medications (such as SSRIs used to treat depression) or other intoxicants (such as MDMA). Both the syndrome and synthetic cannabinoid intoxication can manifest as a fever, a rapid pulse, confusion, and at higher levels can cause organ failure or even death.

As such, it can be hard for emergency medics to work out what treatment a person needs, particularly if they are unable to provide information about what they have consumed, either because they don't know, or because the severity of their intoxication means they cannot communicate it.

Clinicians working with individuals who have used synthetic cannabinoids have noticed an increase in 'stroke-like' presentation at hospitals from people using the substances, due to what are referred to as 'thromboembolic episodes', which refers to when a blood clot or blood clots form in blood vessels – clots then move with the flow of blood, and can block arteries. Hence people being brought into the emergency room with symptoms similar to that of stroke – which is caused by a blockage of the blood flow to the brain.

Synthetic cannabinoid use has been linked to risk of injury to the kidneys, but again, these findings are all from case studies rather than from larger-scale research designs such as cohort studies. All this means that it is hard to say whether these are being caused by the substance itself, or whether the individuals in question have other underlying factors that might also be at play. And given what we know about the people who predominantly use synthetic cannabinoids – in the UK it's largely limited to the prison population and among homeless people – it's plausible that these are groups who are already in poorer health than the general population as a whole.

Any kidney damage or other potential risk factors from synthetic cannabinoids could conceivably be due to other factors related to being homeless or in prison – it is incredibly challenging to unpick. Having said that, the potential link between synthetic cannabinoids and kidney problems is deemed to be important enough that doctors are now advised to consider synthetic cannabinoid use in patients with unexplained acute kidney injury, particularly if they might have other risk factors that would suggest synthetic cannabinoid use.

Stopping using synthetic cannabinoids can be unpleasant. Individuals who use synthetic cannabinoids have reported that they experience comedowns after taking it that can be quite extreme, with symptoms including suicidal ideation – thinking about killing yourself. There is also mounting evidence that synthetic cannabinoids might be more likely to lead to dependence than herbal cannabis. Regular users report experiencing withdrawal symptoms, some of which are similar to those reported by heavy users of herbal cannabis – things such as lack of appetite, feeling irritable, and inability to sleep well.

However, some of the withdrawal symptoms reported by synthetic cannabinoid users are more severe – for example agitation, anxiety, and even seizures. This is another reason that treatment services can struggle to treat people who use synthetic cannabinoids.

Myths and misconceptions

Despite synthetic cannabinoids not having been around for very long, there are already a number of myths and misconceptions that exist around them.

Synthetic cannabinoids are just cannabis that's been made in a factory rather than grown

While synthetic cannabinoids and the naturally occurring cannabinoids found in herbal cannabis both have an effect on the endocannabinoid system in our brains and bodies, this doesn't mean that they're the same compounds. Broadly, synthetic cannabinoids do mimic the effect of THC, the most widely researched cannabinoid that is found in herbal cannabis, and at a molecular level they often look quite similar to THC. However, a slight variation in a molecule can cause a profound change in intoxication effects.

In particular, there's evidence to suggest that the way in which synthetic cannabinoids interact with receptors in the brain is different to that of cannabinoids found in herbal cannabis. THC, in herbal cannabis, is what's known as a partial agonist of cannabinoid receptors in the brain. This means that when THC binds to receptors, it activates or increases activity at that particular site in the brain – but only to a partial degree, and not fully.

Many synthetic cannabinoids are full receptor agonists, meaning they have a much stronger effect at a cellular level in the brain, leading to differences in activation of neural pathways in the brain, different levels of neurotransmitters being present in the gaps (synapses) between neurons, and therefore having dissimilar – stronger – effects.

Not only that, but some synthetic cannabinoids also bind to a variety of other, non-cannabinoid receptors, which might contribute to some of their other reported behavioural and physiological effects. So, while synthetic cannabinoids might be based on herbal cannabis, their effects are usually much more extreme, and unpleasant.

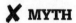 MYTH

Synthetic cannabinoids are safer than cannabis because they are legal

This one flips the usual 'it's natural so it's safer' myth on its head. Some individuals are – perhaps unsurprisingly – swayed by a substance's legal status, assuming this must bear some relation to risk from consuming it. As can be seen from all the descriptions in this chapter, while we know less about the effects of synthetic cannabinoids than we do about herbal cannabis, all the evidence to date suggests that the risk of harm from synthetic cannabinoids is likely to be substantially higher than for herbal cannabis. Not only that, but there are further risks due to how synthetic cannabinoids are prepared.

As I mentioned earlier in the chapter, synthetic cannabinoids are often sprayed onto plant matter to allow them to be smoked. This is a pretty imprecise method of distribution of a substance, and as such, what can happen is that some pieces of plant matter can become super-strength, while others might have almost no psychoactive substance on them at all. This can make judging a dose extremely difficult, above and beyond the usual challenges of not knowing for sure what you are purchasing or consuming when you buy an illicit substance.

There are no regulations controlling production of these substances, and they are often prepared by people without training, in unsafe or unhygienic locations. Even before synthetic cannabinoids were restricted by law, they were always marketed as products that were not safe for human consumption. And the harms from synthetic cannabinoids have increased with each 'generation' created.

Synthetic cannabinoids were originally created as scientific research tools to aid understanding of the endocannabinoid system in relation to factors ranging from brain function to appetite, immune function or psychiatric disorders. The potential for intoxication was not a primary research interest. However, once synthetic cannabinoids began to be made by underground chemists, the intoxication potential was prioritised. Products around at the moment are much more potent, and therefore harmful, than they were in the early 2000s when synthetic cannabinoids first started to be sold.

It's also worth reiterating that 'legal highs' were never really legal – although the products were able to be sold legally for a time, this was only if they were clearly marked as 'not for human consumption'. Legal never meant regulated, and it certainly never meant safe.

 MYTH

Spice makes you a zombie

In the UK there have been many headlines over recent years where synthetic cannabinoids have been held up as causing 'zombie-like' states in people who use them. These stories often focus on people who are homeless, who are highly visible in city and town centres, and who might be attracted to using synthetic cannabinoids in order to cope with the realities of living in the streets. It's been particularly striking in Manchester in the north-west of England, and Wrexham in Wales, among other places.

It's certainly the case that synthetic cannabinoids can induce symptoms that make it difficult to move, or difficult to sit upright. But referring to people as zombies is hugely dehumanising. You wouldn't see headlines referring to people so intoxicated on alcohol that they couldn't stand as zombies, so what is different about synthetic cannabinoids? Perhaps it is the group of people who are using it?

In the UK, the number of people who are homeless has increased dramatically over recent years. Homeless people are often dehumanised and even demonised by the media and authorities, and the attitudes of the general public towards people who are homeless is sometimes less than compassionate. We are advised not to give homeless people money, for example, although this is not based on any evidence.

While synthetic cannabinoids might induce severe intoxication effects, and to see someone standing immobile or slumped in a busy city centre can look strange and disturbing, perhaps it is not surprising that people living in extremely challenging and unpleasant circumstances seek out intoxication that can lead to feelings of dissociation and depersonalisation. And these people should be offered support rather than being dehumanised to the point of referring to them as undead.

The words and phrases that we use to describe other people can lead to stigmatisation and exclusion, and this can have a real impact on public attitudes and the health and safety of targeted groups – research has shown that when more stigmatising terms are used to describe people who use drugs, these people are then more likely to be perceived as having brought their current situation upon themselves, and people are more likely to endorse punitive responses rather than health-based responses.

Certainly, people who use synthetic cannabinoids have been subject to dehumanising treatment. In the UK there have been attacks on individuals who have used synthetic cannabinoids – attacks that have been filmed and put on social media. Sheffield Council issued a statement calling for people to stop posting pictures and videos online. On Facebook, an event calling for 'Spice Zombie bashing' in Doncaster was created and widely shared. This abhorrent behaviour is cruel, and will certainly not help anyone who is probably already struggling.

 MYTH

Do synthetic cannabinoids have any medical uses?

Synthetic cannabinoids were first developed by researchers, and perhaps this makes some sense, given how many illnesses that herbal cannabis has been purported to be able to prevent, treat or cure. Scientists and pharmaceutical companies have been interested in whether cannabinoids can be synthesised that might have the beneficial effects, while minimising the psychoactive or negative side-effects.

Synthetic cannabinoids were investigated as potential treatments for pain, neurodegenerative diseases, and even cancer. For example, the drug nabilone is a synthetic cannabinoid that is used to treat patients with chemotherapy-induced nausea and vomiting. However, most that were created had too many undesired side-effects and were discontinued, only to be picked up by underground chemists and synthesised for recreational use. Once this occurred, the psychoactive effects were prioritised, meaning the most potent compounds were the most popular.

CHAPTER 24

Synthetic Cathinones: Mephedrone and more

MEPHEDRONE

MDPV

What are they? Synthetic substances designed to mimic cathinone – the active compound in khat.

Type of drug: Stimulant.

Popularity: Had widespread media attention in 2000s.

How consumed: Swallowed, or sometimes snorted. Occasionally injected.

Some effects: Euphoria, increased alertness, sociability, insomnia, agitation, heart palpitations, seizures.

SOMETIMES CALLED BATH salts, or plant food, synthetic cathinones were part of the group of novel psychoactive substances (NPS) that appeared in the 1990s and 2000s. They caused a furore in the British and US press – being blamed for everything from cannibalism to genital self-mutilation (more on both of these later).

The compounds themselves are not new; mephedrone and MDPV (two of the most commonly encountered synthetic cathinones) were first recorded in 1929 and 1967 respectively. However, reports of intoxication or abuse of the substances did not occur until much more recently, the 1990s and 2000s – when the substances began to be sold online as 'legal'* alternatives to MDMA or cocaine.

What are they?

Cathinone is the active compound in khat – and so synthetic cathinones are broadly similar compounds, and all are slightly different from cathinone at the molecular level. Some that are particularly common or well-known include mephedrone (4-methyl methcathinone), MDPV (methylenedioxypyrovalerone), flephedrone (4-FMC), 4-bromomethcathinone (4-BMC), ethylone (MDEC), buphedrone, and methylone, to name a few. Phew.

They are known colloquially by a variety of different euphemisms including M-CAT, plant food, bath salts, monkey dust, or meow-meow (this term seemed particularly common in the UK media a few years ago, although whether it was actually used by people who took it is debatable).

Despite each synthetic cathinone being unique at a molecular level, they are hard to distinguish from each other by eye. In fact, they look indistinguishable from many other stimulants; usually found as a white or off-white powder, or more rarely as a tablet or liquid. They are often consumed by snorting, or by wrapping some powder in a cigarette paper and swallowing (bombing). It's uncommon, although possible, to inject them. This method of consumption, though rare, occurs more generally in certain specific groups of people – often among those who inject other substances as well.

---

* Once again, consumption of these substances was never legal – they still had to be marketed as 'not for human consumption' in order to be sold.

Although never legally sold as a product for human consumption, synthetic cathinones were often erroneously known as legal highs. And this might explain some of their appeal; some may have believed that they were safer than drugs such as cocaine or MDMA. In actual fact, even before being brought under criminal law, these products were never under the strict regulation that drugs such as alcohol and tobacco were under. Marketed online as 'plant food' or 'bath salts', there was no regulation or quality control in order to ensure that what you were buying was what it was claimed to be, and as such, mephedrone and the like were just as unknown a quantity as MDMA or cocaine.

What are the short-term effects?

The intoxication effects of synthetic cathinones are similar, although not identical, to the intoxication effects of MDMA, amphetamines or khat. Different synthetic cathinones also have slightly distinctive intoxication profiles from each other, due to their minor chemical differences at the molecular level. For example, MDPV is particularly potent, needing smaller doses to induce intoxication, and therefore also lower doses to experience negative consequences from over-consumption, and risk of toxicity. A number of synthetic cathinones have a relatively short intoxication effect – around two to four hours if swallowed.

Positive effects of synthetic cathinone intoxication can include euphoria, increased alertness, empathy, openness, talkativeness, an increased enjoyment of music and increased sociability, among others. It's probably why synthetic cathinones seem to be popular at raves, parties and festivals, where these substances are likely to be available. They also have a growing popularity among the individuals using them, and other substances, to enhance sexual behaviour, often referred to as 'chem-sex'.

Like other stimulants, synthetic cathinones can reduce appetite, and can also cause insomnia. Higher doses of synthetic cathinones can induce agitation – this is a common symptom reported by individuals who have consumed too much of the substance if they present at hospital or ring services such as the UK's poison information service. Synthetic cathinones can increase blood pressure, and can cause heart palpitations, chest pains, seizures, and hypertension as dose increases. Seizures seem particularly prevalent in children and young adults who have taken large doses of the substances. There have been reports of synthetic cathinone intoxication causing psychosis-like symptoms.

There is some evidence from self-reports that mephedrone is particularly associated with an increased enjoyment of music, or an increased desire to move or dance, compared to other synthetic cathinones. MDPV has been linked to what have been termed 'bizarre behaviours', as well as hallucinations, suicidality and something known as 'excited delirium syndrome' – a set of behaviours somewhat similar to some reports of PCP intoxication, including erratic behaviour, increased strength, a risk of violence, and extremely high body temperature.

Synthetic cathinone intoxication can also cause blurred vision, hot flushes, and muscle tension in the face and jaw similar to that experienced during amphetamine intoxication, due to gurning. If snorted, the substances can lead to irritation of the nasal passages, throat and mouth, and potentially increase the risk of nose bleeds.

Synthetic cathinones have been linked to a likelihood of engaging in risky sexual practices – for example, a study in Ireland asked twenty-two individuals who used mephedrone about how they believed intoxication impacted on their sex lives. They found evidence linking mephedrone intoxication to sexual behaviours including multiple partners and lack of condom use, as well as disinhibition and promiscuity. But they are also linked to chem-sex – the use of drugs, often at parties, to enhance sexual experiences.

Synthetic cathinones (and other substances such as methamphetamine) are reportedly being injected during sex – a behaviour known as 'slamming'. Again, risky sexual practices are more common in these settings, meaning there is an increased risk of blood-borne diseases including HIV and hepatitis B and C from both injecting and from unprotected sex. How common 'slamming' is, it is very hard to ascertain. Evidence thus far has come from very small sub-groups of men who have sex with men in London, and in some French cities, so the true scale of the behaviour is unclear.

Injecting synthetic cathinones conveys a much higher risk of harm, as you would expect. This seems to be a growing problem as well among homeless individuals in Hungary, some of whom are shifting from using heroin to injecting mephedrone. Researchers in Hungary found that people injecting synthetic cathinones were more likely than those using heroin to inject more frequently (some reports from Hungary and Romania suggest up to six or even eleven times a day among some individuals), and to share injection equipment – increasing the risk of blood-borne diseases. More frequent injection also increases the risk of skin and vein damage, abscesses, gangrene, and infections.

Symptoms of synthetic cathinone comedown include low mood, panic attacks, paranoia and in severe cases symptoms of psychosis, which can potentially last for several days, according to a study conducted in Germany that used data from psychiatric inpatient units. There is a small amount of evidence (although it's growing) that MDPV in particular might induce psychological dependence in heavy regular users, and this is backed up by reports from people who use synthetic cathinones regularly of them experiencing withdrawal symptoms when they stop using it, and developing tolerance to it, as well as experiencing craving.

Myths and misconceptions

In the 2010s, the media and the public in the UK and USA in particular were becoming aware of a new substance that was sweeping the streets. The scale of use was hugely exaggerated, and a number of myths and misconceptions sprouted up. Here are a few of the more sensational ones.

Bath salts will turn you into a cannibal

This was based on a story from the USA – on a May 2012 afternoon in Miami, Florida, a naked, thirty-one-year-old man attacked and maimed a sixty-five-year-old man so severely it left him blind in both eyes – the assailant was shot dead at the scene when he ignored police calls for him to stop attacking the man. Eye-witnesses and video footage of the event showed that Rudy Eugene, the attacker, was biting the older man's face. The attack was widely reported, and Eugene was dubbed 'the Causeway cannibal' by the press, because of the location of the attack on Miami's MacArthur Causeway.

News reports stated that Eugene was high on synthetic cathinones at the time of the attack, and that 'bath salts' were responsible for turning him into a cannibal, or zombie. In fact, toxicology reports on Eugene found no suggestion that he had taken synthetic cathinones before the attack. Cannabis was found in his system, and some newspaper reports suggested that there were undigested tablets found in his stomach during the autopsy, which were never identified (although this wasn't reported everywhere, so it's hard to know how accurate this report is).

Either way, 'bath salts' were blamed for the attack without any evidence that they were involved, and the tests done did not find any evidence that they had been consumed. There's never been any other evidence that would suggest synthetic cathinones could make someone exhibit cannibalistic behaviour.

 MYTH

Mephedrone killed two boys in Scunthorpe

In March 2010, two teenage boys died in Scunthorpe, an industrial town near Hull in the north-east of England. Louis Wainwright was eighteen, and his friend Nicholas Smith was nineteen. It was widely reported that they had taken mephedrone, called meow-meow in the press, and died because of it. A media outcry in the UK followed, and mephedrone was banned by the government the following month. However, toxicology reports on the two young men found no mephedrone in their systems.

They had consumed alcohol, and methadone – the substance prescribed to individuals as a substitute for heroin. Methadone and alcohol both depress breathing, and the combination of the two was deemed to be the cause of death for both young men at separate inquests. Whether they were trying to buy mephedrone but had been misled by similar names is unclear, but they had not taken mephedrone on the night they died.

 MYTH

Synthetic cathinones will make you rip your testicles off

'Legal Drug Teen Ripped His Scrotum Off' ran a 2009 headline in the *Sun* newspaper. The story, taken from a police report, claimed that a young man had taken mephedrone and experienced an intense hallucinatory experience, believing himself to be covered with biting centipedes, and needing hospital treatment after ripping his testicles off. Was there any truth to this?

The police report that the story was taken from was an internal memo, and the officer who wrote it stated very clearly in the report that this was information gleaned from online forums – in this case a website about mephedrone – and therefore should be read with that in mind, as there was no evidence to back this story up. *New Scientist* magazine investigated the story further, and the owner of the website reportedly told them that the tale had been uploaded as a joke, to see if the media would bite. And bite they did.

 MYTH

Addiction

One of the biggest fears, individually and societally, from the use of drugs is the risk of addiction. The term 'drug addicts' is a stigmatising title often applied to anyone who uses a drug, but is this fair, or even accurate?

In order to answer that question, we really need to define what we mean by addiction. Colloquially we often use the term addiction to mean 'really liking to do something'. I'm addicted to this new computer game, or I have a chocolate addiction. But when researchers or clinicians speak about addiction, they mean something a little more specific.

Broadly speaking, a behaviour could be considered to be an addiction when an individual changes their life to fit around the consumption of a particular drug. It's not necessarily the quantity of the drug consumed, or even the regularity of use that would define a problem, but the way that use impacts on your life.

Two people could drink the same amount of alcohol and find it impacts on their life in completely different ways. And what changes a compulsion into an addiction is the potential for the compulsion to cause an individual harm. Without this harm, if a person is regularly or heavily using a substance, you might say they had a dependency on it, or potentially not even that – maybe they simply get enjoyment from regular use of it. Of everyone who tries a drug, from coffee to heroin, LSD to cannabis, MDMA to alcohol, many, if not the majority of people will not become addicted to it.

This is even true of heroin, a substance where many think that addiction is inevitable. Addiction rates are hard to estimate, although they seem to be higher than for many other substances, but still lower than most people would estimate if asked. Of course, there are other harms from heroin than just addiction, but the myth that you only need to try it once to become dependent on it is simply not true.

There is only one substance where a large majority of people who try it will go on to develop addiction. And that is tobacco – specifically cigarettes, where a recent systematic review suggested that around 60 per cent of individuals who try a cigarette will become daily smokers, even if only for a short amount of time.

Caffeine is also a substance where the majority of people who use caffeine regularly will experience withdrawal when they stop. Although whether this is truly addiction is contested, as caffeine does not cause harm, or certainly not to the same degree as cigarettes, alcohol or heroin, and therefore it may be more accurate to say people have caffeine dependence.

Perhaps these substances have a higher level of dependence because they are legal and therefore easily available, although the same is true for alcohol, where addiction does occur, but not to such a high degree – around 15 per cent of drinkers will develop problematic alcohol use behaviours.

Why do some people become addicted to substances?

It used to be thought that addiction, or certainly drug dependency, was fairly straightforward. A person used a substance repeatedly, and their body and/or brain became tolerant to the substance, requiring more and more of it to maintain function. This concept of addiction suggested that treatment was simple – stop taking the substance, and allow the brain and body to return to their pre-addicted state. But there are several ways in which this is over simplistic. For a start, it doesn't explain why some people (the majority of people, in fact) can use a substance and not develop addiction.

We know a bit about how drugs affect the brain – they impact on the chemicals that transmit signals between brain cells – the neurotransmitters. Some have suggested that addiction might develop because substances alter the chemical balance of our brain by impacting on these neurotransmitters. Potentially, regular consumption of a substance that mimics a specific neurotransmitter might lead to the brain creating or releasing less of it, which could be unpleasant, and lead an individual to take more of the drug to 'top up' their levels.

One neurotransmitter in particular has been associated with addiction: a chemical called dopamine. There is a pathway within our brains often referred to as the dopamine reward pathway, and activation through this path is linked to, as you might guess, reward, as well as things like pleasure and enjoyment. As such, this pathway is strongly linked to addiction, and is often seen activated or implicated in brain-scan studies of people with drug dependence. But it's also been shown to be linked to other things we might really enjoy doing, such as eating delicious food, watching our favourite TV show, or having sex.

Are we addicted to these things? I'd argue not, apart from in extremely rare cases, suggesting that dopamine and the dopamine reward pathway's involvement might be a little more nuanced than we think. It seems like there's something else above and beyond brain chemical changes that leads to addiction.

The bio-psycho-social model of addiction

A landmark study that has influenced theories of addiction was conducted by Lee Robins, a psychiatric epidemiologist from Louisiana, USA. It was well-documented that American troops in Vietnam showed unusually high levels of drug use while deployed. In particular, they were using heroin or opium, with around 35 per cent of US soldiers using heroin, and 20 per cent showing signs of dependence on it.

Robins followed up a group of veterans when they returned from Vietnam to the USA in 1971, and found that although some continued to use drugs on their return (around 10 per cent reported having used heroin in the eight to twelve months since they returned from Vietnam), the vast majority stopped using heroin as soon as they were back in their home communities, and fewer than 1 per cent of her sample reported becoming re-addicted after returning home. This study implied that a person's circumstances can strongly impact on their ability to avoid (or succumb to) addiction.

Robins didn't stop at collecting the numbers, she also asked the men in her sample why they didn't carry on using heroin once they had returned to the USA. Most reported that it was easy to obtain it where they lived, but they did not continue to use it because of factors such as fear of addiction, disapproval of family and friends, and fear of arrest. This certainly supports the idea that the environment in which they found themselves, a war zone far from home, versus their own community, was able to override any biological impact of the substance.

Robins' work strongly supports a model of addiction where the substance is important, but so is the environment a person is in, their personal circumstances, and even their personality. This is known as the bio-psycho-social model of addiction, stressing the importance of biology, psychological factors and social circumstance. This model suggests that some people are likely to be particularly vulnerable to developing dependence, for a variety of reasons. And this is backed up by research evidence.

Likelihood to experience addiction runs in families – if your parents or siblings struggle with their substance use, you are more inclined to as well. This may be genetic, or could be environmental, and in reality is probably a bit of both. Socio-economic status also predicts risk of addiction. If your life is more challenging, maybe you're more likely to use a substance to cope with that, which can lead to problematic use. Or perhaps people from higher socio-economic backgrounds are still experiencing problems, but can better access support and treatment due to their circumstances.

Personality-wise, impulsivity seems to be linked to a risk of developing problematic substance use, but as with all these factors, it is not necessary or sufficient. Each of these factors might tip the scales, and there are probably a load of other risk factors for addiction that we're not aware of yet.

A similar finding is that of Rat Park. Rat Park was an experiment conducted in the late 1970s in Canada by a man called Bruce K. Alexander. At this time, most research into models of addiction was conducted on rodents. For the most part, these animals were kept isolated, in small cages, and researchers such as Alexander were beginning to wonder whether the lack of environmental stimulation might be impacting on the research.

The way the findings of Rat Park are presented in popular culture often goes something like this:

Alexander found that rats in cages in his psychology department would self-administer morphine at high levels. The rats were kept in small metal cages, isolated from each other and from pretty much any stimulation at all – the only thing they really saw were the psychologists who fed them, and occasionally made them do a water maze or some other experiment. So Alexander built 'Rat

Park', a large cage complex where multiple rats were housed, with room to roam, levels to explore, and all manner of stimulation. He found that rats in this environment were far less likely to self-administer morphine, and were more likely to drink plain water.*

However, when you go back to the original Rat Park papers, published between 1978 and 1981, the story is a little less dramatic. While Alexander and his co-authors did indeed find a difference in morphine-laced water consumption between the rats in Rat Park and those in isolated cages, this was only in very specific circumstances.

Firstly, in the initial study, the rats in all conditions barely touched the morphine-water to begin with. In order to get them to consume it, they were all given no choice but to consume it – their other water was taken away for over fifty days. This part of the experiment was so extreme that four female rats died during it – two who were in Rat Park, and two who were in isolation. This left a very small sample size indeed – only two females and six males were left in isolation, and eight females and twelve males in Rat Park.

The two isolated females consumed way more morphine water than any of the other groups of rats, driving the difference between isolation and Rat Park. There were some other slightly strange things about the way the experiment was run as well. The way water and morphine consumption was measured was different between the two groups. In Rat Park a complicated system involving cameras and laser beams was set up. In isolation, the rats' water bottles were weighed at the beginning and end of each

---

* This is actually a quote from myself – I wrote this in the proposal for this very book. Since then, I have written an article for the journal *Addiction*, as part of their Classics series, about Rat Park, which led me to thoroughly read the original papers. I was quite shocked at just how different the public perception of the research is from what Alexander and his colleagues actually did.

day. If there was some systematic difference in error rate between these two ways of measuring, that would show a difference even if one didn't exist.

The fact that the difference was particularly striking in the female rats may also be important. Rats in Rat Park weren't separated by sex. As such, it's extremely likely that there were rat babies. The pregnancy and weaning of rat pups may have impacted on the female rats in Rat Park's behaviour, making them less comparable to those in isolation.

All this isn't to say that the findings of Rat Park aren't important. Many other studies have also found that environment – set and setting – can have a big impact on these kinds of animal studies, and it's widely accepted that this bio-psycho-social model of addiction, where biology, psychology and social setting all impact on a person's likelihood to develop problematic substance use, is important to understanding human behaviour.

But as is so often the case when studies like Rat Park seem to be *Just So* stories – if it seems as if the findings are too good to be true, they probably are.

Stigma

There's another factor that might make addiction more difficult for an individual, and harder to break out of, and that's stigma. There's an alarming amount of evidence that suggests that drug use is something viewed as immoral and deviant by large swathes of the planet. This is true individually, and at governmental (and higher) levels.

When the United Nations published their international treaty in 1961, the Single Convention on Narcotic Drugs, they referred to addiction to drugs as 'a serious evil' for the individual, and 'fraught with social and economic danger to mankind'. Quite extreme language. India's supreme court went further still in 2003, declaring that offences related to drugs were worse than murder 'because the latter affects only an individual while the former affects . . . society, besides shattering the economy of the nation'.

Surveys conducted across the world have shown that people often have negative views of those who use substances. In 2016, a survey conducted in Scotland on public attitudes towards people with drug dependence found that 42 per cent of respondents believed that drug dependence was due to a lack of self-discipline and willpower – pinning the blame firmly on the individual.

Research conducted in North Africa and the Middle East asked individuals to describe people who inject drugs. The most commonly used terms in response were 'should be punished', 'evil/mean persons', 'disrespected/disrespectful', 'guilty'. A 1998 USA survey asked people to select words or phrases that described a person who uses cocaine. The most commonly selected were 'no future', 'lazy', and 'self-centred'.

How we refer to someone impacts on how they are perceived and treated, even among healthcare professionals who might be those to whom these individuals would go for help.

A study in the USA gave mental health clinicians a vignette about a person – but these vignettes were slightly tweaked. Some people read vignettes with neutral language, while others read about 'addicts' who were 'problem drug users'. Where the language used was more pejorative, these clinicians were more likely to believe that the individual was responsible for their situation. Not only that, but they also endorsed more punitive measures towards the individual. So while it might seem awkward or unnecessarily PC to use overly long descriptions such as 'people who inject drugs' or 'people with problematic substance use' rather than terms like junkie or addict, it's really important to do so.

Language matters, and there's a real risk that individuals who do experience problems with their substance use will be less likely to seek help, or get the help they need, if they're stigmatised for their situation.

Nobody starts using drugs with the intention of becoming addicted or dependent on them. And while, as indicated by both Rat Park and the Vietnam Veterans study, a person's circumstances can increase the risk that occasional use will turn into regular use, and in turn on to problematic use and potentially addiction, there are other factors at play.

Equally, while we know that certain brain regions play a role in addiction and addictive behaviours, presenting addiction as purely a brain disease might be counter-productive. It could imply to those who are beginning to move down this path towards problematic use that there's little they can do about it, which might lead to feelings of helplessness, and an inability to take action to improve.

Although conversely, it could give those who believe they don't have an 'addictive personality' a false sense of security about their drug taking, as they might believe themselves immune to the risk of dependence.

Risk factors for addiction are both nature and nurture – it is likely that some people have a higher innate risk of developing addiction, based on their genetic makeup. But if they never try a substance, this increased risk won't have any effect. Similarly, lots of environmental influences can play a role – a difficult childhood, trouble at work or at home, all sorts of things. But plenty of people will really struggle in their lives, and not then develop problems with drug use.

It is complicated, and at the moment while we know at a population level some of the factors that increase the risk of addiction, we can't predict which individuals will develop dependence, or addiction.

Drug Use in
the Real World

This book is about the science of various different substances. It's about what we know (and don't know) about the chemical compound MDMA and its effects on people, or heroin, or any other substance detailed within these pages.

But drug use, particularly illicit drug use, does not necessarily follow these neat classifications. If you buy a white powder, or a chalky tablet, from someone you know, from a stranger at a festival, even over the internet, you are really buying a lottery ticket. There are no consumer rights for illicit drugs.

While pharmaceutical substances have to be created under very strict conditions, in sterile environments, and to high quality standards, illicit drugs that are synthesised or even just packaged in underground labs are subject to none of these. They may be prepared by amateurs, in bulk, in unhygienic or dirty environments. And there's absolutely no guarantee that what you're purchasing contains what you think it does, or doesn't contain something else that could potentially cause you unexpected harms, or a dose far greater than what you're expecting.

While each chapter in this book focuses predominantly on the harms from a specific known substance, it's vital to be aware that there are additional risks when a person takes a powder, a tablet or a liquid. There are specific things that people who decide to take a drug can do to minimise these harms, although as we've said throughout this book, no drug use is without harm.

Is it the substance you think it is?

A white powder or a non-descript tablet could contain many things. Unfortunately, there is no way to be fully sure that what you're taking is what you think it is. This can put people at serious risk of harm. As an example, in the early 2010s, a substance called PMA was being sold in the UK and around Europe as MDMA, and it put seasoned MDMA users in danger. PMA takes longer than MDMA for intoxication to begin. Not only that, but it has a smaller window of efficacy – you only need to take slightly more of it to tip from the sought-after intoxication experience into overdose and unpleasant or dangerous toxicity.

People who were used to taking MDMA would take PMA, wait until they expected to feel something, then, assuming they had a low-potency batch of MDMA, take more, and push themselves into toxicity. Although PMA is less commonly being sold as MDMA nowadays, these types of substitutions are common, and have happened with MDMA throughout its illicit history.

The Drug Policy Alliance report on their website that 'MDMA' has been found containing synthetic cathinones, amphetamine, cocaine, caffeine, and less commonly ketamine or dextromethorphan, an ingredient found in cough medicines. One online drug-testing company published data on MDMA samples sent to them in 2015. Of 250 samples, 124 did not contain MDMA, and forty contained MDMA and one of the substances mentioned above.

This is not only a problem for MDMA. Heroin has been tested and found to be laced with the substantially more potent opioid fentanyl. There is no way to tell this by looking at the sample, and if a person injected what they thought was a standard dose of heroin, they would be at high risk of severe harm or even death from fentanyl overdose. Fentanyl has also been found disguised as the benzodiazepine Xanax.

There are things you can do to reduce the risk from unknown substances. It is possible to buy drug-testing kits online, but these will test only for specific substances – if the powder or tablet contains anything else it won't pick this up, and it might not be able to tell you about the strength of the dose either. In recent years, and in certain countries, drug testing on-site at music festivals, or in city centres, is beginning to become more common, although at the time of writing this is still quite rare.

These services can not only provide information to individuals, but can also provide public information, for example about high-potency tablets in local circulation, or adulterated pills that contain harmful unexpected substances. However, even these sites – particularly when in the (festival) field – can only test for certain contents, and will not necessarily be able to tell you every single substance in your powder or tablet.*

Is it the dose you think it is?

As has been detailed in some of the specific chapters in this book, a powder or a tablet can hide secrets about the concentration of the substance it contains, even if it is what you think it is. This is also the case for substances where the psychoactive compound has been sprayed onto plant-based material, and even substances like cannabis, where the levels of THC can vary dramatically between different plants, and different preparations of cannabis.

---

* They'll be able to tell you exactly what they can and can't tell you about your sample, should you have the need to use their services.

Not only that, but a suitable dose of any substance is a very individual matter – affected by your genetics, your biological sex, what you've eaten that day, even your mood. This can be clearly seen with alcohol – if I tried to drink ten pints I would be extremely ill, whereas some of my friends can do this easily and even be able to function adequately the next day.

There are steps that you can take to avoid the risk of over-dosing on a substance. The first is to try what is called titration. This means starting with a very low dose, and gradually increasing the dose until you find a point where the sought-after effects outweigh the unwanted side-effects. This is how doctors might work out a correct dose of medication – and it's far less risky than just starting with a dose you think might work and hoping for the best.

If you're taking a powder or pill, harm-reduction advice is to 'crush dab wait', which means taking a small amount of powder or crushed pill and dab a licked finger into it, take that and wait for an hour or two before deciding whether to take more. This advice was in response to high-purity MDMA crystals being in circulation, which people were consuming whole and experiencing unpleasant intoxication or overdose symptoms.

Another slogan is 'don't be daft, start with a half', which concerns MDMA tablets. In recent years these have been increasing in potency, some being found to contain four times the level found in tablets a decade ago.

Taking illicit drugs is more dangerous today than it's ever been

While I was finalising the edits to this book, in August 2019, the UK's Office for National Statistics published their latest report about drug-related deaths in England and Wales – the deaths reported in 2018 where drugs were mentioned on the death certificates. And it made for pretty sobering reading. Drug poisoning deaths are at the highest levels they have been since the data started being collected in 1993. ONS reported that 4,359 individuals died in 2018 due to drug poisoning in England and Wales.

In particular, there were rises in deaths from people using cocaine (the data combined powder cocaine and crack cocaine), opioids (in particular heroin and morphine), amphetamine, and benzodiazepines. The National Crime Agency reported that cocaine that has been seized recently is at what they described as 'historically high' purity levels, which could be one explanation for why deaths from cocaine have increased substantially.

The drug death situation is even worse in Scotland, where 1,187 deaths were reported last year, ranking it as a country with one of the highest rates of drug-related deaths globally. The reasons why drug deaths are increasing are likely to be complicated, relating to purity, the closure of drug-treatment and support services, austerity politics, and all sorts of other factors. Public Health England have identified risk factors for drug-related deaths, which include people who use many different drugs (and alcohol), people who consume drugs while they are alone, and people who live alone.

What can be done? The research community in the UK was quite vocal about this in the wake of these figures being published: harm-reduction strategies need to be prioritised, funding that has been cut to support services needs to be reinstated, and consideration of the complex needs of the people most at risk from drug-related death needs to be at the forefront of any policies.

This is only likely to happen with public support, but drug use, and particularly drug dependence, is still heavily stigmatised. The more we can humanise people who use drugs, the more compassionate we can be, the more likely we are to see a change in how people are treated, and hopefully a change in the direction of the ONS's graphs.

Many people reading this book will be doing so out of curiosity, and will perhaps have tried one or two of the substances I've described. I would not encourage anyone to take any of the substances mentioned here. No drug use is without risk of harm. This is true of illicit drugs, and it is true of licit ones.

I'm sure some people reading this are parents, concerned as to what is out there that their child might be tempted to try. For you, I hope this book can help you to start conversations that can be based on evidence-based information and the principles of harm reduction.

Some people will have picked up this book because they have tried many of the substances detailed within its pages. For you, I hope that you have found it an interesting trip.

Glossary

These are some of the terms and concepts that I talk about throughout the book, with a little more detail about what I mean by them.

Absolute risk – the probability that an event will occur. For example, how likely you are to develop bowel cancer (around 5 per cent of the population will get this cancer at some point in their lives). This is in contrast to a **relative risk**, which is the difference in probability depending on a certain characteristic. For example, how likely you are to develop bowel cancer if you eat a lot of processed meat compared to people who eat none (you're 21 per cent more likely to develop bowel cancer). Relative risk can sound quite scary – 21 per cent increased risk sounds like a lot! But given the absolute risk is low, it's actually only a small increase in real terms. The absolute risk of bowel cancer for people who eat a lot of processed meat is 6 per cent, one percentage point higher than for those who don't.

Anaesthetic – a medication (drug) that is used to induce temporary unconsciousness (in the case of a general anaesthetic), or numbness (local anaesthetic) in the individual it is given to. Similar is a **sedative**, a drug used to induce calm or sleep in an individual, but not necessarily unconsciousness or a lack of ability to feel pain.

Central nervous system (CNS) – in humans (and in fact all vertebrates) the brain and spinal cord. This is the part of the nervous system that controls the body – receiving information from the rest of the body and processing and responding to it.

Cognition - the act of learning or thinking. Cognition refers to any brain process involved in thought, knowledge or skill. Examples of cognitive processes include attention, perception, memory, learning, language, and higher reasoning processes such as **executive function**.

Confounding – in an observational study, individuals are observed doing what they would usually do, rather than being randomly assigned to a condition, as would happen in an **RCT**. There are going to be differences other than those that you're interested in, and these are the **confounders**. An observational study should therefore take account of these confounders in its statistical analysis, as otherwise an analysis might just show the impact of these differences on your outcome of interest, rather than the exposure you are interested in. As an example – there is a strong association seen between sales of ice cream and incidences of skin cancer. There is **confounding** affecting this association, and the confounder that is likely to be particularly important is sunny weather.

Depersonalisation – a feeling or sensation of being separate or detached from yourself. It might feel like you're looking at yourself from outside your body, or it might feel like you're detached from your emotions, or have a sense that you're not yourself. Also related is **derealisation** – the feeling of detachment or separation from the world around you, or a feeling that people or things are not real.

Dissociative (e.g. dissociative anaesthetic) – dissociation is the act of feeling separate or disconnected from your surroundings. **Depersonalisation** or **derealisation** might be symptoms of dissociation. A dissociative anaesthetic is a drug that induces an inability to move, memory loss, and a lack of ability to move, as well as feelings of detachment or separation from the world.

Double blind – a way of designing a research study. In a double-blind study, neither the participant nor the researcher know whether the individual has been put in the experimental or control group of the study – for example, whether they are being given a drug or a placebo. The reason for designing studies in this way is that people can be tricksy when you try and research them – hoping to please the experimenter, whether intentionally or unintentionally. Knowing what experimental condition they're in could impact on how they report their symptoms. But this can also be true of experimenters themselves. If experimenters know who is in what condition, they might notice positive symptoms more easily in the experimental condition, even if they don't realise that's what they're doing. Not knowing who's in which condition takes away this risk of bias.

Drug – a substance that is consumed, that impacts on the body or the brain in some way. This could include medications, prescribed for all sorts of physical or mental ailments, or substances consumed because of potential pleasurable effects to the individual. Of course, some substances could fall into both these categories.

Epidemiology – a field of research concerned with investigating health and disease at a population level. Often using large datasets, it looks for patterns in the data as to how prevalent certain illnesses or health behaviours are, what predicts health or illness, and evidence for what interventions could improve health outcomes. Epidemiology is considered a part of medicine, is taught to medical students, and is usually seen as part of Social Medicine or Public Health research.

Executive function – a term that covers higher-level cognitive processes, specifically those related to carrying out behaviours. These are the processes required to plan and execute goal-related behaviours. This includes working memory (holding things in short-term memory), inhibitory control (the ability to withhold a response on command), fluid intelligence (reasoning and problem-solving skills), the ability to switch between multiple tasks, and these kinds of processes.

Genotype – the genetic makeup of an individual. Each person has two copies of their genetic material, half from their biological mother, and half from their biological father. The genotype is the combination of both sets of genetic material, meaning everyone has two copies of every gene, of every chromosome (apart from the sex chromosomes, where – mostly – females have two Xs, and males have an X and a Y).

Intoxication – the psychoactive effects of a substance. The 'high', or the 'trip'. Being drunk on alcohol is an example of an intoxication experience. Some people use the term intoxication to refer specifically to the experience of taking too much of a substance, and the unpleasant effects that can arise, but in this book, I am using the term to refer to the pleasant and unpleasant effects of consuming a drug.

Molecule – a group of atoms that are connected in a specific way by chemical bonds. Also the smallest unit of a particular compound (H_2O is a molecule of water – two hydrogen atoms bonded to one oxygen atom).

Neuron – a brain cell. A long, thin cell that transmits signals along its length via electrical impulse.

Neurotransmitter – a chemical found in the brain (and elsewhere in the body) that passes signals across the gaps between brain cells (neurons). Examples of neurotransmitters include dopamine, serotonin, GABA and endorphins.

Phenotype – the observable characteristics of an individual, as a result of the combination of their genotype and their environmental influences. For example, your height, hair, skin and eye colour, personality type and your behaviours (whether or not you use alcohol, or you like coffee), would all be part of your phenotype, and considered phenotypic traits.

Placebo – a substance, or a treatment, which is designed to look like an experimental substance or treatment, but actually has no therapeutic value. I won't say 'has no effect', because there have been many studies conducted that show that a placebo treatment can lead to some level of improvement for a number of conditions. Once again, humans are tricksy – in much the same way that set and setting can have an influence on intoxication, being given a treatment can impact on symptoms, even if the treatment is nothing more than a sugar pill, an injection of saline solution, or a sham therapy of some kind. Exactly why the placebo effect occurs is not very well known, but it has been consistently shown.

Psychopathology – the study of mental ill health and mental disorders.

Psychopharmacology – the study of the impact of drugs on mind and behaviour. From psychology and pharmacology.

Psychosis – a mental disorder where individuals perceive things that are not there. This often takes the form of hallucinations, seeing or hearing things that are not there, and delusions, believing something about oneself that is not true. A **psychotic episode** is a period of time where a person experiences these symptoms, which is often extremely distressing for them and those around them. Psychosis or psychotic episodes are some of the symptoms of schizophrenia – though not all people with schizophrenia will have psychosis, and not everyone who experiences a psychotic episode will be diagnosed with schizophrenia.

Randomised controlled trials (RCTs) – a way of designing a research study, or trial (the T of the RCT). If you're interested in the effect of x on y, you might take a group of people, randomly (the R . . . you get the gist) split them to either receive x or to not receive x (called a control group, the C of the RCT), and follow them up to see how many who were given x develop y, and how many who were controls develop y. This method of conducting a study is sometimes called, rather grandly, the gold standard of **epidemiological** research. And it is a good way of answering a number of health-related questions, particularly if the design can be double-blind too. However, there are some health questions where an RCT is not possible. Sometimes this is for a practical reason – if you're interested in the impact of an exposure over a long period of time, months or years (as you often are when thinking about the risks of regular use of a drug), then RCTs are impractical. They would be too expensive, and it would be very hard to keep people compliant with the experimental condition they were put in.

Set and setting – this is the idea that where you are, and how you're feeling will influence an intoxication experience. There's quite a lot of evidence to back up the importance of mood and environment, but as to why they are so important, that's less well understood. But who you're with, where you are, and how you're feeling are all likely to impact on how pleasant or unpleasant any intoxication experience you have might be.

Synaesthesia – a condition where individuals experience links or connections between two (or more) senses that are usually separate. For example, noises may elicit tastes, or music might elicit an experience of seeing colours. Many synaesthetes do not realise they have synaesthesia until they learn about it, potentially not realising others do not experience the world in the same way as them. Synaesthesia is not considered an illness and most people with it find it enhances their experience of the world, rather than detracting from it. However, some individuals with certain types of synaesthesia can find it impairing, for example where numbers appear coloured, this can interfere with ability to perform maths. Others find that their synaesthesia can improve their abilities, for example memory can be enhanced for some synaesthetes.

Synapse – the gap between two (or more) **neurons** (brain cells). Human brain cells are very long and thin – some stretch up to a metre in length. Where a neuron ends, many arms extend out of it, called dendrites. These dendrites brush up close to other neurons – in fact each neuron can be connected to up to 10,000 other neurons! But they don't touch each other, and the gap between them is called a synapse. Neurons communicate via electrical impulses that travel along the length of the neurons. These impulses can't travel across the synapses, so when the electrical impulse reaches the end of each dendrite, it triggers the release of chemicals called **neurotransmitters** across the gap (called, rather sexily, the synaptic cleft). These neurotransmitters travel across the gap and bind to receptors in the next neuron, allowing the electrical impulse to then continue its journey.

Window of efficacy – sometimes known as the therapeutic index, this is the dosage range in which a drug will have the desired effect. Below this range, the drug is likely to be ineffectual, and above this range the drug may be toxic and pose a risk to health or potentially even to life.

Acknowledgments

To Doug and Iggy, to my Mum and Dad, Sarah, and all my family and friends, thank you for your unerring support, and for always making me feel like nothing is impossible.

Thanks to my *Guardian* science blog pals, in particular Alok, James (R and K), Tash, Pete, Chris, Dean and Martin, and to Dylan and Neil with whom I first set up a science blog.

Huge thanks to Scroobius Pip. He took a chance inviting me on his podcast back in 2015, and became the catalyst in getting *Say Why to Drugs* the podcast off the ground. I think it's unlikely you'd be reading this book today if Pip hadn't got involved, and offered me so much support and encouragement over the years. I'm hugely grateful to Adam Richardson and Charlie Williams for their invaluable help making *SWTD* look and sound better than I ever could have. Thanks to acast for hosting the podcast, and to the rest of the Distraction Pieces extended network, Stu, Chris, Jason, Brett, Matt, Jim, Dan, John, Warren, for being such a blummin nice bunch of blokes.

Thank you to the fantastic colleagues I have had past and present, TARG in Bristol, and the Appetite and Addiction group in Liverpool. And to Praveetha, for her excellent counsel and creative vision while I've been writing.

Thanks to my PhD supervisors Stan Zammit, Matt Hickman, Jon Heron and Marcus Munafo, for instilling in me a love of this topic, a love of critical thinking and for helping me learn the skills to synthesise evidence.

On countless occasions I have thrown questions I've been struggling with to Twitter, and drug science and drug policy tweeps have been incredibly helpful when I've been looking for errant stats or miscreant references – thank you all.

Huge thanks to my incredible agent Kate, whose encouragement, constructive comments and support through the book-writing process has been invaluable. And to my brilliant editor Huw for his enthusiasm and championing. To my fellow Wellcome Trust Engagement fellows for helping me expand my thinking, and to the BSA and BBC science unit where I undertook a Science Media Fellowship, thank you.

A number of experts have lent their time to read over some of the chapters in this book, explain nuanced findings to me, or otherwise offer advice. I'd like to thank Sally Adams, Peter Rogers, Jasmine Khouja, Carl Roberts, Abi Rose, Olivia Maynard, Linda Bauld, Valentina Lorenzetti, Danny Chambers, Kevin Fong, Jason Reed, Shalini Arunogiri, Albert Garcia-Romeu, Matt Kennelly, Oliver Grundmann, Tim Williams, Hazel Phillips, Kate Flemming, Celia Morgan, Amir Englund, Matt Hickman and Abu Shafi for their thoughtful comments. Their kindness, generosity with their time, and their insightful peer review have markedly improved the book. I owe a particular debt of gratitude to Harry Sumnall, who has offered me thoughtful and knowledgeable advice for many years, and in particular for this book.

Thanks also to the people who spoke candidly to me about their drug use, and provided the quotes in this book. I haven't named you here, but you know who you are.

Thank you to Neko Case, Marika Hackman and Nadine Shah for writing amazing albums that have kept me company while writing.

I'm sure there are many other brilliant people I have forgotten to name personally, and I apologise – if you should be on this list but aren't, thank you, and forgive me!

This book wouldn't be half what it is without these people, but any mistakes that remain are mine and mine alone.

References and Further Reading

General

When I first started making my podcasts, as well as looking at recently published research, I found Professor David Nutt's book *Drugs Without the Hot Air*, published by UIT Cambridge, extremely useful. The organisation David set up, Drug Science, has an excellent website drugscience. org.uk, which has evidence-based information about a number of different substances.

For practical advice about minimising the risks if you are planning to take an illicit substance, the website drugsand.me offers practical advice for before, during and after a trip.

If you're interested in a bit more of the molecular science of various substances, *The Drug Classroom* on YouTube is a great resource.

And if it's policy that you're interested in, you can't go wrong with the excellent 'Stop and Search' podcast, published on the Distraction Pieces Network (the same as Say Why to Drugs), and created by Jason Reed at LEAP UK, an organisation of individuals who have previously worked in law enforcement, and are now against prohibition.

A lot of the figures about substance use, misuse, and deaths came in England and Wales came from the Office for National Statistics' website. Their reports are very clearly written and worth a look if you're interested in patterns of data over recent years and decades. European stats come from the European Monitoring Centre for Drugs and Drug Addiction website, a fantastic resource. The EMCDDA have also written excellent individual substance profiles, a number of which were used as source material for the book. I've also reported some stats from the Global Drugs Survey, and their website has a number of interesting reports on substance use patterns.

Alcohol

Terry Mulhern, 'Why do people with East Asian heritage get flushed after drinking alcohol?', December 27 2017, The Conversation website.

Some of the hangover papers I discuss:

Kochling et al. 'Grape or grain but never the twain? A randomized controlled multiarm matched-triplet crossover trial of beer and wine'. 2019, *The American Journal of Clinical Nutrition*.

Rohsenow and Howland. 'The role of beverage congeners in hangover and other residual effects of alcohol intoxication: a review'. 2010, *Current Drug Abuse Reviews*.

If you're interested in the science of hangovers, the work of Dr Sally Adams is worth exploring. Sally Adams, 'The Science of Hangovers', December 19 2013, *The Guardian*. And her meta-analysis investigating the effect of hangover on cognition is published Gunn et al. 'A systematic review of the next-day effects of heavy alcohol consumption on cognitive performance', 2018, *Addiction*.

James Morris. 'The media has a problem with alcoholism – and it's stopping people getting help'. November 22 2017, *The Guardian*.

Julie Corliss. 'Is red wine actually good for your heart?' February 19 2018, Harvard Health Blog.

This is a great article discussing the evidence linking alcohol to poor (or good) health, and the strength of it, by my stats hero, David Spiegelhalter. Everyone has a stats hero, right?

David Spiegelhalter, 'The risks of alcohol (again)', August 24 2018, The Winton Centre on Medium.

Neuroskeptic, 'The Myth of Beer Goggles?', August 20 2015, *Discover Magazine*.

This article investigates how attractive individuals are rated before and after they have consumed alcohol:

Van Den Abbeele et al. 'Increased Facial Attractiveness Following Moderate, but not High, Alcohol Consumption'. 2015, *Alcohol and Alcoholism*.

Mamluk et al. 'Low alcohol consumption and pregnancy and childhood outcomes: time to change guidelines indicating apparently "safe" levels of alcohol during pregnancy? A systematic review and meta-analyses'. 2017, *BMJ Open*.

Amphetamine

Some fascinating blogs exploring the history of amphetamine use:

Jesse Hicks, 'Fast Times: The Life, Death, and Rebirth of Amphetamine, Distillations Magazine', April 14 2012, Science History Institute.

Erin Blakemore, 'A Speedy History of America's Addiction to Amphetamine', October 27 2017, *Smithsonian Magazine*.

Neurofantastic, 'The Rainbow Diet Pills: There and Back Again', June 22 2014.

Here is a list of some of the other articles I used as source material for the chapter.

A couple of papers about the history of amphetamine:

Rasmussen. 'America's First Amphetamine Epidemic 1929–1971: A Quantitative and Qualitative Retrospective With Implications for the Present'. 2008, *American Journal of Public Health*.

Heal et al. 'Amphetamine, past and present – a pharmacological and clinical perspective'. 2013, *Journal of Psychopharmacology*.

This paper explores the impact of amphetamine on brain structure:

Berman et al. 'Abuse of amphetamine and structural changes in the brain'. 2008, *Annals of the New York Academy of Sciences*.

This is the paper that looked at the dental health of people who use various different drugs:

Laslett et al. 'The oral health of street-recruited injecting drug users: prevalence and correlates of problems'. 2008, *Addiction*.

This paper discusses the use of amphetamines for treating ADHD:

Brown et al. 'Pharmacologic management of attention deficit hyperactivity disorder in children and adolescents: a review for practitioners'. 2018, *Translational Pediatrics*.

Jeanette Wick, 'Recreational Drug Use: A Risk Factor For Glaucoma?', May 23 2012, *Pharmacy Times*.

Dr Shalini Arunogiri wrote this review exploring the evidence linking amphetamine use and psychosis:

Arunogiri et al. 'The Methamphetamine-Associated Psychosis Spectrum: a Clinically Focused Review'. 2018, *International Journal of Mental Health and Addiction*.

Luke Williams, 'The Speed You're Taking Is Probably Just Meth', July 26 2016, *VICE*.

Benzodiazepines

Some history:

Sujata Gupta. 'Mother's Little Helper: A brief history of benzodiazepines'. March 17 2015. *Mosaic Science*.

Jeanette Wick. The History of Benzodiazepines. 2013, *The Consultant Pharmacist* (article and podcast).

The annual report of WEDINOS, the Welsh postal drug testing service:

PHILTRE, Annual Report 1st April 2017 – 31st March 2018, Harm Reduction Wales. Wales NHS.

Noel Philips. '"Xanax" linked to more than 200 deaths', February 5 2019. BBC News website.

These pages from the USA's National Institute for Health website detail research investigating the co-use of benzodiazepines and opioids, and potential risk factors associated:

National Institute on Drug Abuse. 'Benzodiazepines and opioids'. Revised March 2018, Drugabuse.gov website.

Here are a couple of papers exploring the (weak) evidence for valarian to treat anxiety and insomnia:

Miyasaka et al. 'Valerian for anxiety disorders'. 2006, *Cochrane Systematic Reviews – Intervention*.

Leach M., and Page, A. 'Herbal medicine for insomnia: A systematic review and meta-analysis'. 2015, *Sleep Medicine Reviews*.

This report is a little old, but details what was known about the potential risks of using benzodiazepines during pregnancy:

McElhatton. 'The effects of benzodiazepine use during pregnancy and lactation'. 1994, *Reproductive Toxicology*.

Caffeine

If you're interested in finding out more about caffeine, I really enjoyed reading Murray Carpenter's book *Caffeinated*, published in 2014 by Hudson Street Press.

Hourglass PJ, 'Caffeine in your drink: Natural or synthetic?' May 2 2012, *The Pharmaceutical Journal* blog.

Durlac. 'A rapid effect of caffeinated beverages on two choice reaction time tasks'. 2002, *Nutritional Neuroscience*.

Luis Villazon, 'How long does caffeine take to kick in?'. *Science Focus Magazine*.

This is the study that went to cafes across Europe and examined the caffeine content in espressos:

Ludwig et al. 'Variations in caffeine and chlorogenic acid contents of coffees: What are we drinking?' 2014, *Food and Function*.

University of Florida, 'Decaffeinated coffee is not caffeine free, experts say'. October 15 2006, *Science Daily*.

Joe Watts, 'Government to introduce energy drinks ban for teenagers and children'. August 30 2018, *The Independent*.

European Food Safety Authority, 'Caffeine: EFSA estimates safe intakes'. May 27 2015.

This blog has detailed cases where caffeine has been implicated in fatalities:

Caffeine Informer, 'Documented Deaths by Caffeine', CaffeineInformer.com

Franziska Spritzler, '9 side effects of too much caffeine'. August 14 2017, Healthline.com

Ding et al., 'Long-Term Coffee Consumption and Risk of Cardiovascular Disease: A Systematic Review and a Dose–Response Meta-Analysis of Prospective Cohort Studies'. 2014, *Circulation*.

Casey Dunlop, 'Coffee and cancer – what does the evidence say?' June 15 2016, Cancer Research UK Science blog.

Michelle Z. Donahue, 'Do you love or loathe coffee? Your genes may be to blame'. November 2 2018. *National Geographic*.

Here are a couple of Peter Rogers' papers and articles I mention in the chapter:

Rogers et al. 'Faster but not smarter: Effects of caffeine and caffeine withdrawal on alertness and performance'. 2013, *Psychopharmacology*.

'Coffee consumption unrelated to alertness'. June 2 2010, University of Bristol press release.

This paper reviews the link between coffee use and health, with a critical eye:

James. 'Are coffee's alleged health protective effects real or artifact?

The enduring disjunction between relevant experimental and observational evidence'. 2018. *Journal of Psychopharmacology*.

Fukimaki et al. 'Serum caffeine and metabolites are reliable biomarkers of early Parkinson disease'. 2018, *Neurology*.

Cannabis

Steve Fiorillo. 'What's the difference between indica vs. sativa?' July 2 2019. *TheStreet*.

D'Souza et al. 'The psychotomimetic effects of intravenous delta-9-tetrahydrocannabinol in healthy individuals: implications for psychosis'. 2004, *Neuropsychopharmacology*.

Zhang et al. 'Cannabis smoking and lung cancer risk: Pooled analysis in the International Lung Cancer Consortium'. 2015, *International Journal of Cancer*.

Gage et al. 'Association between cannabis and psychosis: Epidemiologic evidence'. 2016, *Biological Psychiatry*.

Meier et al. 'Persistent cannabis users show neuropsychological decline from childhood to midlife'. 2012, *PNAS*.
    Mokrysz et al. 'Are IQ and educational outcomes in teenagers related to their cannabis use? A prospective cohort study'. 2016, *Journal of Psychopharmacology*.

The Mistaking Histories blog picks apart the 'Queen Victoria used cannabis' claim in great detail here:
    'Queen Victoria's cannabis habit: again'. August 29 2017. Mistaking histories blog.

McGuire et al. 'Cannabidiol (CBD) as an adjuctive therapy in schizophrenia: A multicenter randomized controlled trial'. 2018, *American Journal of Psychiatry*.

This paper asked individuals in Netherlands who used cannabis about their preference for THC and CBD in the cannabis they are using:

Schubert. 'Cannabis with high cannabidiol content is associated with fewer psychotic experiences'. 2011, *Schizophrenia Research*.

Alexandra Jones, 'Cannabis has been given a chic rebrand. But are the (legal) products worth it?' November 2018. *Stylist Magazine*.

Smart et al. 'Variation in cannabis potency and prices in a newly legal market: Evidence from 30 million cannabis sales in Washington state'. 2017, *Addiction*.

Chandra et al. 'New trends in cannabis potency in USA and Europe during the last decade (2008-2017)'. 2019, *European Archives of Psychiatry and Clinical Neuroscience*.

Budney et al. 'An update on cannabis use disorder with comment on the impact of policy related to therapeutic and recreational cannabis use'. 2019, *European Archives of Psychiatry and Clinical Neuroscience*.

Evidence for the effectiveness of CBD for epilepsy is gathered on the website for the charity Epilepsy Action.

Cigarettes

The World Health Organisation has excellent infographics about the history of tobacco on their website. There is a lot of information about the harms of smoking on the Cancer Research UK web pages.

Young et al. 'Prevalence and attributes of roll-your-own smokers in the International Tobacco Control (ITC) four country survey'. 2006, *Tobacco Control*.

Edwards. 'Roll your own cigarettes are less natural and at least as harmful as factory rolled tobacco'. 2014, *BMJ Personal View*.

Brennan et al. 'Tobacco particulate matter self-administration in rats: differential effects of tobacco type'. 2013, *Addiction Biology*.

Leavell. 'The low tar lie'. 1999, *Tobacco Control*.

Jarvis and Bates. 'Why low tar cigarettes don't work and how the tobacco industry has fooled the smoking public'. 1999, Action on Smoking and Health website.

Suzi Gage. 'Hooked on Shisha: Why hookahs might be more harmful than you think'. April 19 2016. *The Guardian*.

Gage and Munafo. 'Rethinking the association between smoking and schizophrenia'. 2015, *Lancet Psychiatry*.

Hart et al. 'Genetic correlation between smoking behaviors and schizophrenia'. 2018, *Schizophrenia Research*.

Cocaine

Patrick Barkham. 'Cocaine in rivers harming endangered eels, study finds'. June 21 2018. *The Guardian*.

Emily Goddard. 'Why so many young Brits are smoking crack'. March 5 2018. *VICE*.

Anna Pursglove. 'The cocaine hypocrisy: This is who's really buying drugs in the UK'. June 2019. *Stylist Magazine*.

This blog details the use of coca leaves to manage altitude sickness, and the practice of mixing coca leaves with lime:
'Coca leaf as a travel necessity'. November 4 2014. Panaceachronicles blog.

Jamie Doward. 'Warning of extra heart dangers from mixing cocaine and alcohol'. November 8 2019. *The Guardian*.

Anna Codrea-Rado. 'Is coke vegan? And other urban drug myths busted'. November 20 2018, BBC Three.

Mayukh Sen. 'Is cocaine vegan? It depends on who you ask'. November 29 2017. *VICE*.

National Institute on Drug Abuse. 'What are the effects of maternal cocaine use?'. Revised May 2016, Drugabuse.gov website.

De Giorgi et al. 'Cocaine and acute vascular diseases'. 2012, *Current Drug Abuse Reviews*.

Here's a selection of interesting articles about the history of cocaine:
    Mikkel Borch-Jacobsen. 'Ernst Fleischl von Marxow (1846-1891): Freud's first therapeutic blunder and how he lied about it'. February 7 2012. *Psychology Today*.
    Howard Markel. 'Cocaine: A Brief History of Blow'. CBS News.
    'Cocaine'. Updated August 21 2018. History.com

DMT

A lot of the source material for this chapter came from the book *DMT: The Spirit Molecule*, by Rick Strassman, published by Inner Traditions Bear and Company.

Benjamin Taub. 'Do our brains produce DMT, and if so, why?' July 5 2017, Beckley Foundation blog.

Nichols. 'N,N-dimethyltryptamine and the pineal gland: Separating fact from myth'. 2017, *Journal of Psychopharmacology*.

E-cigarettes

There is a lot of clear information about e-cigarette research and evidence on the *Action on Smoking and Health* (ASH) website, including a number of fact sheets about issues such as youth use of e-cigarettes.

Linda Bauld and Suzi Gage. 'Vaping by young people remains a burning issue among health experts'. January 4 2019, *the Guardian*.

Kim Lacapria. 'Vaping causes "Popcorn Lung"?' August 8 2016, Snopes.com

'Does vaping cause popcorn lung?' Reviewed October 19 2018, Cancer Research UK website.

Here are some papers and reports exploring whether or not e-cigarette use might be linked to pneumonia:
Miyashita et al. 'E-cigarette vapour enhances pnuemococcal adherence to airway epithelial cells'. 2018, *European Respiratory Journal.*
'E-cigarettes may make lungs vulnerable to infection'. Feburary 5 2015. NHS Behind the Headlines webpages.
Campagna et al. 'Respiratory infections and pneumonia: Potential benefits of switching from smoking to vaping'. 2016, *Pneumonia.*

'Smoking still a leading cause of fatal fires warns Brigade on No Smoking Day'. March 14 2018, London Fire Brigade website.

Lion Shahab and his colleagues investigate the different impacts of NRT, e-cigarettes and cigarettes on levels of various carcinogens and toxins, in this research:
Shahab et al, 2017. 'Nicotine, Carcinogen, and Toxin Exposure in Long-Term E-Cigarette and Nicotine Replacement Therapy Users: A Cross-sectional Study'. *Annals of Internal Medicine.*

Yuan et al. 'Nicotine and the adolescent brain'. 2015, *Journal of Physiology.*

The Truth Initiative published a list of the way e-cigarettes might harm the environment on their website. Healthon's comment piece discusses the environmental harm from cigarettes:
'3 ways JUUL harms the environment'. April 23 2019, Truth Initiative website.
Healton et al. 'Butt really? The environmental impact of cigarettes'. 2011, *Tobacco Control.*

GHB

For advice about GHB, what it is, and reducing the risks if you plan to use it, there is excellent information on the Terrence Higgins Trust web pages. The Turningpoint.org.au Australian website has advice for individuals seeking to reduce or stop their use of GHB.

This article goes in depth into the science of GHB, GBL and 1,4-butanediol:

Wood. 'Gamma-hydroxybutyrate and its related analogues gamma-butyrolactone and 1,4-butanediol'. 2017, *Critical Care Toxicology*.

These papers compile the evidence linking GHB to sexual assaults:

Nemeth et al, 2010. 'Review: The involvement of gamma-hydroxybutyrate in reported sexual assaults: a systematic review'. *Journal of Psychopharmacology*.

Butler and Welch. 'Dug-facilitated sexual assault'. 2009, *CMAJ*.

Dick Talens. 'Bodybuilders and using roofies to work out. Wait, what?' November 19 2015, Thrillist website.

This paper explores whether and why GHB might be found naturally occuring in the body:

Elian, 2002. 'Determination of endogenous gamma-hydroxybutyric acid (GHB) levels in antemortem urine and blood'. *Forensic Science International*.

Kamal et al. 'The neurobiological mechanisms of gamma-hydroxybutyrate dependence and withdrawal and their clinical relevance: A review'. 2016, *Neuropsychobiology*.

Heroin

Ciccarone. 'Heroin in brown, black and white: Structural factors and medical consequences in the US heroin market'. 2010, *International Journal of Drug Policy*.

The stat that 23 per cent of opioid users develop dependence comes from this report:
'Opioid addiction 2016 Facts and Figures'. *American Society of Addiction Medicine*.

However, a number of other researchers dispute these figures, for example:
Sweeting et al. 'Estimating the prevalence of ex-injecting drug use in the population'. 2008, *Statistical Methods in Medical Research*.

Hickman et al. 'Estimating the relative incidence of heroin use: Application of a method for adjusting observed reports of first visits to specialized drug treatment agencies'. 2001, *American Journal of Epidemiology*.

Editorial. 'Opioids and methamphetamine: a tale of two crises'. 2018. *The Lancet*.

Gossop and Strang. 'A comparison of the withdrawal responses of heroin and methadone addicts during detoxification'. 1991, *British Journal of Psychiatry*.

If you are interested in finding out more about drug consumption rooms, the website of the International Network of Drug Consumption Rooms has a lot of information about them.

Ketamine

These papers are an excellent starting point if you're interested in a synthesis of the scientific evidence around ketamine:
Morgan et al. 'Ketamine use: a review'. 2012, *Addiction*.
Taylor et al. 'Ketamine – the real perspective'. 2016. *Lancet*.
The World Health Organisation has a fact file about ketamine on their website.

John Hamilton. 'Ketamine, a promising depression treatment, seems to act like an opioid'. August 29 2018. *NPR Shots*.

'Ketamine tested as severe depression treatment'. April 3 2014. NHS Behind the Headlines webpages.

'Ketamine has "fast acting benefits" for depression'. April 16 2018. BBC News website.

Clark. 'Veterinary use of ketamine'. British Association for Psychopharmacology web pages.

'The dangers of equine anaesthetics'. September 16 2005, *Horse and Hound* magazine.

Joel Frohlich. 'Schizophrenia in a vial? The story of ketamine'. September 19 2017, *Psychology Today*.

Liu et al. 'Ketamine abuse potential and use disorder'. 2016, *Brain Research Bulletin*.

This paper explores how acute doses of ketamine impact on individuals who are given it in the lab:

Pomraol-Clotet. 'Psychological effects of ketamine in healthy volunteers: Phenomenological study'. 2006, *The British Journal of Psychiatry*.

This lab study shows that ketamine might encourage neuronal growth in rats:

Yang et al. 'Acute administration of ketamine in rats increases hippocampal BDNF and mTOR levels during forced swimming test'. 2013, *Upsala Journal of Medical Science*.

This is the reference for the study that investigated the impact of cutting down ketamine use on a variety of outcomes:

Morgan et al. 'Beyond the K-hole: a 3-year longitudinal investigation of the cognitive and subjective effects of ketamine in recreational users who have substantially reduced their use of the drug.' 2004, *Addiction*.

This research found nasal administration of ketamine to show low tolerability and not to be a useful treatment:

Galvez et al. 'Repeated intranasal ketamine for treatment-resistant depression – the way to go? Results from a pilot randomised controlled trial'. 2018. *Journal of Psychopharmacology.*

This pilot trial, from the Black Dog Institute in Australia, found promising results for the treatment of depression in elderly patients – although it was a very small-scale study:

George et al. 'Pilot randomized controlled trial of titrated subcutaneous ketamine in older patients with treatment-resistant depression'. 2017, *The American Journal of Geriatric Psychiatry.*

Khat

This paper explores the evidence linking khat use and dental problems, particularly cancer:

Math and Kattimani. 'Khat and cancer'. 2016, *British Dental Journal.*

Nigussie et al. 'Association between khat chewing and gastrointestinal disorders: a cross sectional study'. 2013, *Ethiopian Journal of Health Sciences.*

Odenwald et al. 'Khat use as a risk factor for psychotic disorders: a cross-sectional and case-control study in Somalia'. 2005, *BMC Medicine.*

Kratom

This is the letter to the journal *Addiction* that first sparked my interest in kratom:

Grundmann et al. 'The therapeutic potential of kratom'. 2018, *Addiction.*

This paper is a case study of an individual self-medicating their opioid withdrawal using kratom:

Boyer et al. 'Self-treatment of opioid withdrawal using kratom (Mitragynia speciosa korth)'. 2008, *Addiction.*

Grundmann. 'Patterns of kratom use and health impact in the US – results from an online survey'. 2007, *Drug and Alcohol Dependence*.

Singh et al. 'Changing trends in the use of kratom (Mitragyna speciosa) in Southeast Asia'. 2017, *Human Psychopharmacology*.

This paper explores some of the case studies where kratom has been associated with psychosis symptoms:

Bestha. 'Kratom and the opioid crisis'. 2018, *Innovations in Clinical Neuroscience*.

This paper details a case study where an individual using kratom developed jaundice:

Kapp et al. 'Intrahepatic cholestasis following abuse of powdered kratom (Mitragyna speciosa)'. 2011, *Journal of Medical Toxicology*.

These blogs all discuss the current legal status of kratom in the USA, and controversies surrounding it:

Sessi Kuwabara Blanchard. 'Ohio plans to ban kratom – and the DEA may be close behind'. October 12 2018, *Filter* magazine.

Larry Greenemeier. 'Should kratom use be legal?' September 30 2013, *Scientific American*.

Troy Farah. 'The U.S. may ban kratom? But are its effects deadly or lifesaving?' November 15 2018, The Crux blog, *Discover Magazine*.

LSD

A lot of the source material for this chapter, particularly the historical details and quotes, and details of the short-term drug effects, were taken from Albert Hofmann's excellent autobiography:

LSD My Problem Child, translated by Jonathan Ott, and published by Beckley Foundation Press. I also read and enjoyed John Higgs' I Have America Surrounded—a book detailing the life of Timothy Leary and the adventures in psychedelic research.

De Gregorio et al. 'Chapter 3 – D-Lysergic acid diethylamide, psilocybin, and other classic hallucinogens:

Mechanism of action and potential therapeutic applications in mood disorders'. 2018, *Progress in Brain Research*.

Here are a selection of papers investigating the impact of LSD on chromosome damage – the original papers purporting a negative effect, and later debunking articles:

Cohen et al. 'The effect of LSD-25 on the chromosomes of children exposed in utero'. 1968, *Pediatric Research*.

Dishotsky et al. 'LSD and genetic damage'. 1971, *Science*.

Lee and Shlain. *Acid Dreams: The complete social history of LSD: The CIA, the sixties and beyond*. 1985, Grove Press.

Kaelen et al. 'LSD enhances the emotional response to music'. 2015, *Psychopharmacology*.

This blog post explores the myth that LSD is stored in fat and could be re-released at any moment to cause a flashback:

Keith Veronese. 'Could you actually have an LSD flashback decades after taking the drug?' October 19 2012, Gizmodo website.

These articles detail information about grapefruit juice and why it is risky to take alongside some medications:

Vu. 'Grapefruit juice and some oral drugs: A bitter combination'. 1999, *Nutrition Bytes*.

'Grapefruit juice and some drugs don't mix'. July 18 2017, U.S. Good and Drug Administration website.

The MAPS website details their ongoing research looking at psilocybin and LSD, as well as some published research, including:

Gasser et al. 'Safety and efficacy of lysergic acid diethylamide-assisted psychotherapy for anxiety associated with life-threatening diseases'. 2014, *The Journal of Nervous and Mental Disorder*.

Ian Sample. 'LSD's impact on the brain revealed in groundbreaking images'. April 11 2016, *The Guardian*.

Carhart-Harris et al. 'Neural correlates of the LSD experience revealed by multimodal neuroimaging'. 2016, *PNAS*.

Kevin Franciotti. 'We're starting to understand how psychedelic flash-backs work'. May 19 2017, *VICE*.

Here are a number of articles about microdosing, which highlight a) how popular articles about it are, and b) how little research there currently is:

M. Tabu. 'I microdosed with LSD for a month and this is what it did to me'. October 8 2017, IFLScience website.

Ban Taub. 'Here's why LSD microdosing could be the next major breakthrough in mental healthcare'. April 6 2017. IFLScience website.

Sarah Boseley. '"It lifted me out of depression": Is microdosing good for your mind?' September 1 2018, *The Guardian*.

Yanakieva et al. 'The effects of microdose LSD on time perception: a randomised, double-blind, placebo-controlled trial'. 2019, *Psychopharmacology*.

Liechti. 'Modern clinical research on LSD'. 2017, *Neuropsychopharmacology*.

Nour et al. 'Psychedelics, personality and political perspectives'. 2017, *Journal of Psychoactive Drugs*.

A few papers exploring HPPD:

Halpern and Pope. 'Hallucinogen persisting perception disorder: what do we know after 50 years?'. 2003, *Drug and Alcohol Dependence*.

Orsolini et al. 'The "endless trip" among the NPS users: Psychopathology and psychopharmacology in the hallucinogen-persisting perception disorder. A systematic review'. 2017, *Frontiers in Psychiatry*.

Noushad et al. '25 years of hallucinogen persisting perception disorder – a diagnostic challenge'. 2015, *British Journal of Medical Practitioners*.

This paper gave healthy individuals LSD in the lab, and spoke to them again a year later – they found individuals reported that the LSD experience was a personally meaningful one with long-term positive effects:

Schmid and Liechti. 'Long-lasting subjective effects of LSD in normal individuals'. 2018, *Psychopharmacology*.

MDMA

I really enjoyed this fascinating article about the history of MDMA:
Mike Power. 'Ecstasy island: This is the story of how MDMA reached the UK in 1988'. May 3 2018, *Mixmag*.

Kennedy et al. 'Ecstasy and sex among young heterosexual women: A qualitative analysis of sensuality, sexual effects, and sexual risk taking'. 2010, *International Journal of Sexual Health*.

Daisy Buchanan. 'Leah Betts died 20 years ago and we still can't be honest about drugs'. November 16 2015, *The Telegraph*.

N.B.: THIS ARTICLE HAS BEEN RETRACTED. Ricaurte et al. 'Severe dopaminergic neurotoxicity in primates after a common recreational dose regimen of MDMA ("ecstasy")'. 2002, *Science*.
Rick Weiss. 'Results retracted on ecstasy study'. September 6 2003. *The Washington Post*.

Roberts et al. 'Meta-analysis of executive functioning in ecstasy/polydrug users'. 2016, *Psychological Medicine*.

Roberts et al. 'Meta-analysis of molecular imaging of serotonin transporters in ecstasy.polydrug users'. 2016, *Neuroscience and Biobehavioral Reviews*.
Szigeti et al. 'Are ecstasy induced serotonergic alterations overestimated in the majority of users?' 2018, *Journal of Psychopharmacology*.

Passie. 'The early use of MDMA ("Ecstasy") in psychotherapy (1977–1985)'. 2018, *Drug Science, Policy and Law*.

This blog mentions the MDMA bumper stickers:

Mike Sheffield. 'Could MDMA save your relationship?' February 17 2016, Complex website.

This research looked at whether drug deaths from MDMA were over-reported in the Scottish press:

Forsyth. 'Distorted? A quantitative exploration of drug fatality reports in the popular press'. 2001, *International Journal of Drug Policy*.

Nicole Lee. 'How does MDMA kill?'. January 22 2019, *The Conversation*.

Nitrous oxide

A few articles about the history of nitrous:

Goerig and Schulte am Esch. 'History of nitrous oxide – with special reference to its early use in Germany'. 2001, *Best Practice and Research Clinical Anaesthesiology*.

Boyle. 'Nitrous oxide: History and development'. January 27 1934, *The British Medical Journal*.

Esther Inglis-Arkell. 'The strictly non-medical history of laughing gas'. August 16 2012, *Gizmodo*.

'The wacky history of nitrous oxide: It's no laughing matter'. July 20 2015, DOCS Education website.

Doug Bolton. 'Global Drugs Survey finds that nitrous oxide is the second most popular drug in the UK'. June 8 2015, *The Independent*.

Acharya et al. 'Laughter isn't always the best medicine. Recreational use of nitrous oxide is an emerging public health problem'. 2018, *BMJ Editorial*.

Beth Brockett. 'Greenhouse gas: Why nitrous oxide is no laughing matter for the environment'. January 26 2015, *The Conversation*.

Anil Seth. 'Your brain hallucinates your conscious reality'. April 2017 TED talk.

PCP

A few articles looking at the history of PCP:

Thombs. 'A review of PCP abuse trends and perceptions'. 1989, *Public Health Reports*.

Lodge and Mercier. 'Ketamine and phencyclidine: the good, the bad and the unexpected'. 2015, *British Journal of Pharmacology*.

Domino and Luby. 'Phencyclidine/Schizophrenia: One view toward the past, the other to the future'. 2012, *Schizophrenia Bulletin*.

In this *NY Times* article, a toxicologist is quoted as saying that no PCP was found in the blood samples taken from Rodney King:

'Rodney King testifies about night of beating'. January 22 1993. *The New York Times*.

Big Lurch interview, from the documentary *Rhyme and Punishment*, directed by Peter Spirer, 2009. Uploaded to YouTube January 18 2013 by xXDisco DonutXx.

Dominici et al. 'Phencyclidine intoxication case series study'. 2015, *Journal of Medical Toxicology*.

These articles explore the link between schizophrenia and violence (as an aside, the Mental Elf website is an extremely useful resource to find out more about recently published research around mental health – highly recommended):

Rebecca Syed. 'Are you really at risk of attack by someone with schizophrenia?' June 24 2013, The Mental Elf website.

Varshney et al. 'Violence and mental illness; what is the true story?' 2015, *Journal of Epidemiology and Community Health*.

Is PCP use on the rise? This article explores the question in the USA:

Bush. 'Emergency department visits involving phencyclidine'. 2013, *The CBHSQ Report*.

Poppers

Rewbury et al. 'Poppers: legal highs with questionable contents? A case series of poppers maculopathy'. 2017, *British Journal of Opthalmology*.

Paul Berg. 'Use of "poppers" linked to Kaposi's sarcoma'. April 24 1985, *The Washington Post*.
    Anupriya et al. 'Long-term nitrite inhalant exposure and cancer risk in MSM'. 2017, *AIDS*.

A mouse model paper looking at learning, memory and motor control:
    Cha et al. 'Neurotoxicity induced by alkyl nitrites: Impairment in learning/memory and motor coordination'. 2016, *Neuroscience Letters*.

Oscar Quine. 'Poppers: How gay culture bottled a formula that has broken down boundaries'. January 22 2016, *The Independent*.

A couple of articles about poppers and cyanide poisoning:
    Petrikovics et al. 'Past, present and future of cyanide antagonism research: From the early remedies to the current therapies'. 2015, *World Journal of Methodology*.
    Lavon and Bentur. 'Does amyl nitrite have a role in the management of pre-hospital mass casualty cyanide poisoning?' 2010, *Clinical Toxicology*.

Are poppers psychoactive? A few articles and letters that explore this question:
    Joshua Badge. 'Amyl nitrite: Australia's ban on poppers is an attack on gay and bisexual men'. October 17 2018, *The Guardian*.
    Letter to Karen Bradley MP, Minister for Preventing Abuse, Exploitation and Crime, from Professor Les Iverson (Chair of the Advisory Council on the Misuse of Drugs). 'RE: ACMD review of alkyl nitrites ("poppers")'. Dated 16 March 2016, Accessed via UK government website.
    Alan Travis. 'Poppers escape ban on legal highs'. March 22 2016, *The Guardian*.

Prescription opioids

Katherine Sleeman and John Strang. 'Opioids: Why "dangerous" drugs are still being used to treat pain'. July 22 2018, BBC News website.

'What are opioids and what are the risks?' March 19 2018, BBC News website.

'DrugFacts: What are prescription opioids?' Revised June 2019, National Institute on Drug Abuse website.

'Opioids Aware: A resource for patients and healthcare professionals to support prescribing of opioids medicines for pain'. Faculty of Pain Medicine in partnership with Public Health England (accessed from FPM website).

Associated Press. 'Prescription opioids fail rigorous new test for chronic pain'. March 6 2018, *Stat News*.

Sarah Wakeman. 'Fentanyl: The dangers of this potent "man-made" opioids'. August 5 2016, Harvard Health Blog.

Some articles exploring whether you can overdose on fentanyl just by touching it:

'ACMY and AACT Position Statement: Preventing occupational fentanyl and fentanyl analog exposure to emergency responders'. *American College of Medical Toxicology*.

Maia Szalavitz. 'You can't overdose on fentanyl by touching it'. March 21 2018, *VICE*.

German Lopez. 'You can't overdose on fentanyl by touching it. The myth that you can, however, is genuinely dangerous'. March 22 2019, *Vox*.

Some articles investigating the use of opioids in the UK, the USA and Canada, and how to improve the situation:

Ingrid Torjesen. 'Fentanyl misuse in the UK: will we see a surge in deaths?'. 2018, *BMJ Briefing*.

Sarah Boseley. 'Prescription of opioid drugs continues to rise in England'. February 13 2018, *the Guardian*.

Niko Kommenda et al. 'Why are more Americans than ever dying from drug overdoses?' November 29 2018, *the Guardian*.

'Responding to Canada's opioid crisis'. Modified May 9 2019, Government of Canada's website.

'Opioid overdose crisis'. Revised January 2019, National Institute on Drug Abuse website.

'Oxycodone-with-naloxone controlled-release tablets (Targin) for chronic severe pain'. October 25, 2011, NPS Medicinewise website.

Psilocybin

Some research looking at prevalences of different psychedelics:

Krebs and Johansen. 'Over 30 million psychedelic users in the United States'. 2014, F1000 Research.

Johnson et al. 'Classic psychedelics: An integrative review of epidemiology, therapeutics, mystical experience, and brain network function'. 2019, *Pharmacology and Therapeutics*.

Beug and Bigwood. 'Psilocybin and psilocin levels in twenty species from seven genera of wild mushrooms in the Pacific Northwest, U.S.A.' 1982, *Journal of Ethnopharmacology*.

Lauren Slater. 'Psilocybin could help terminal patients face their fear of death'. April 2018, *Discover Magazine*.

The work by Robin Carhart-Harris and colleagues to look at the impact of psilocybin on the human brain:

Carhart-Harris et al. 'Neural correlates of the psychedelic state as determined by fMRI studies with psilocybin'. 2012, *PNAS*.

Petri et al. 'Homological scaffolds of brain functional networks'. 2014, *Journal of the Royal Society Interface*.

Tia Ghose. 'Magic mushrooms create a hyperconnected brain'. October 29 2014, *LiveScience*.

Garcia-Romeu and Richards. 'Current perspectives on psychedelic therapy'. 2018, *International Review of Psychiatry*.

Lyons and Carhart-Harris. 'Increased nature relatedness and decreased authoritarian political views after psilocybin for treatment-resistant depression'. 2018, *Journal of Psychopharmacology*.

A number of papers that investigated the impact of psilocybin on the brain:

Vollenweider et al. 'Positron emission tomography and fluorodeoxy-glucose studies of metabolic hyperfrontality and psychopathology in the psilocybin model of psychosis'. 1997, *Neuropsychopharmacology*.

Vollenweider et al. 'Psilocybin induces schizophrenia-like psychosis in humans via a serotonin-2 agonist action'. 1998, *Neuroreport*.

Hasler et al. 'Acute psychological and physiological effects of psilocybin in healthy humans: A double-blind, placebo-controlled dose-effect study'. 2004, *Psychopharmacology*.

Salvia

Sumnall et al. 'Salvia divinorum use and phenomenology: results from an online survey'. 2011, *Journal of Psychopharmacology*.

El-Khoury and Sahakian. 'The association of salvia divinorum and psychotic disorders: A review of the literature and case series'. 2015, *Journal of Psychoactive Drugs*.

Susan Donaldson James. 'Salvia studies hold promise for addiction'. January 3 2010. ABC News.

'Miley Cyrus breaks her silence. I'm sorry. I never, ever said I was perfect'. March 2011. *Marie Claire* magazine.

Synthetic cannabinoids

This paper describes a few case studies where synthetic cannabinoid intoxication has presented to hospital as similar to serotonin syndrome:

Louh and Freeman. 'A "spicy" encephalopathy: synthetic cannabinoids as a cause of encephalopathy and seizure'. 2014, *Critical Care*.

Bick et al. 'Synthetic cannabinoid leading to cannabinoid hyperemesis syndrome'. 2014, *Mayo Clinic Proceedings*.

Mensen et al. 'Psychopathological symptoms associated with synthetic cannabinoid use: a comparison with natural cannabis'. 2019, *Psychopharmacology*.

Ashlet Yeager. 'How K2 and other synthetic cannabinoids got their start in the lab'. November 27 2018, The Scientist website.

Tracey et al. 'Novel psychoactive substances: Types, mechanisms of action, and effects'. 2017, BMJ Clinical updates (article and podcast).

Synthetic cathinones

Sam Iravani. 'Health risks associated with mephedrone use: What we know so far'. March 6 2019, Talking Drugs website.

Prosser and Nelson. 'The toxicology of bath salts: a review of synthetic cathinones'. 2012, *Journal of Medical Toxicology*.

Weinstein et al. 'Synthetic cathinone and cannabinoid designer drugs pose a major risk for public health'. 2017, *Frontiers in Psychiatry*.

Assi et al. 'Profile, effects, and toxicology of novel psychoactive substances: A systematic review of quantitative studies'. 2017, *Human Psychopharmacology*.

Van Hour and Brennan. '"Bump and grind": An exploratory study of mephedrone users' perceptions of sexuality and sexual risk'. 2011, Drugs and Alcohol Today.

These papers explore the injecting drug use in Hungary:
    Peterfi et al. 'Changes in patterns of injecting drug use in Hungary: A shift to synthetic cathinones'. 2014, *Drug Testing and Analysis*.

Tarjan et al. 'Emerging risks due to new injecting patterns in Hungary during austerity times'. 2015, *Substance Use and Misuse*.

'Perspectives on synthetic cathinones'. Updated June 4 2015, EMCDDA website.

'Men attending group sex "slam parties" don't all use or inject drugs'. Aids Ark website.

Some articles exploring the media reports linking synthetic cathinones to some outlandish incidents:

Jacob Sullum. 'The legend of the Miami cannibal provides lessons in shoddy drug journalism'. May 5 2016, *Forbes*.

'Teenagers deaths "not caused by mephedrone"'. May 28 2010, BBC News website.

'Scunthorpe community "awash with methadone"'. January 25 2011. BBC News website.

Jane Fae. 'Internet and journos fertilise scrotum-ripping drug panic'. December 2 2009, *The Register*.

Nic Fleming. 'Miaow-miaow on trial: Truth or trumped-up charges?' March 29 2010, *New Scientist*.

Addiction

'Most people who try one cigarette become daily smokers, study says'. January 10 2018, BBC News website.

Hall and Weier. 'Lee Robins' studies of heroin use among US Vietnam veterans'. 2017, *Addiction*.

Gage and Sumnall. 'Rat Park: How a rat paradise changed the narrative of addiction'. 2018, *Addiction*.

'The world drug perception problem. Countering prejudices about people who use drugs'. 2017, Global Commission on Drug Policy.

This paper asked a USA-based sample to select terms to describe an individual who uses cocaine. The results, as they say, may shock you:

Blendon et al. 'The public and the war on illicit drugs'. 1998, *Journal of the American Medical Association*.

Abaza. 'Multicentre Operational Research on Drug Use and Harm Reduction among People living with HIV/AIDS in the Middle East and North Africa Region'. 2017, Beirut: Menahra.

A number of papers that explore the issue of stigma, in various populations:

Kelly and Westerhoff. 'Does it matter how we refer to individuals with substance-related conditions? A randomized study of two commonly used terms'. 2010, *International Journal of Drug Policy*.

Lloyd. 'The stigmatization of problem drug users: A narrative literature review'. 2013, *Drugs: Education, Prevention and Policy*.

McCreaddie et al. 'Routines and rituals: A grounded theory of the pain management of drug users in acute care settings'. 2010, *Journal of Clinical Nursing*.

Henderson et al. 'Social stigma and the dilemmas of providing care to substances users in a safety-net emergency department'. 2008, *Journal of Health Care for the Poor and Underserved*.

Bryan et al. 'Public attitudes towards people with drug dependence and people in recovery'. 2016, the Scottish Government.

Lines, R. '"Deliver us from Evil?" – The Single Convention on Narcotic Drugs, 50 Years On'. 2010, *International Journal on Human Rights and Drug Policy*.

These are the details of the ruling of the India supreme court where they described drug crime as worse than murder:

Pasayat. J.A (2003) 'Union of India vs Kuldeep Singh on 8 December, 2003'.

Who uses drugs in the needle park in Zurich?

Grob. 'The needle park in Zurich: the story and the lessons to be learned'. 1994, *European Journal on Criminal Policy and Research*.

Drugs in the Real World

The Drug Policy Alliance have a number of articles and resources on their website related to this, including one detailing common adulterants found in MDMA. The Loop's website is another excellent resource for evidence-based information.